Echidna with NUT ALLERGY

Understanding FOOD ALLERGY & ANAPHYLAXIS

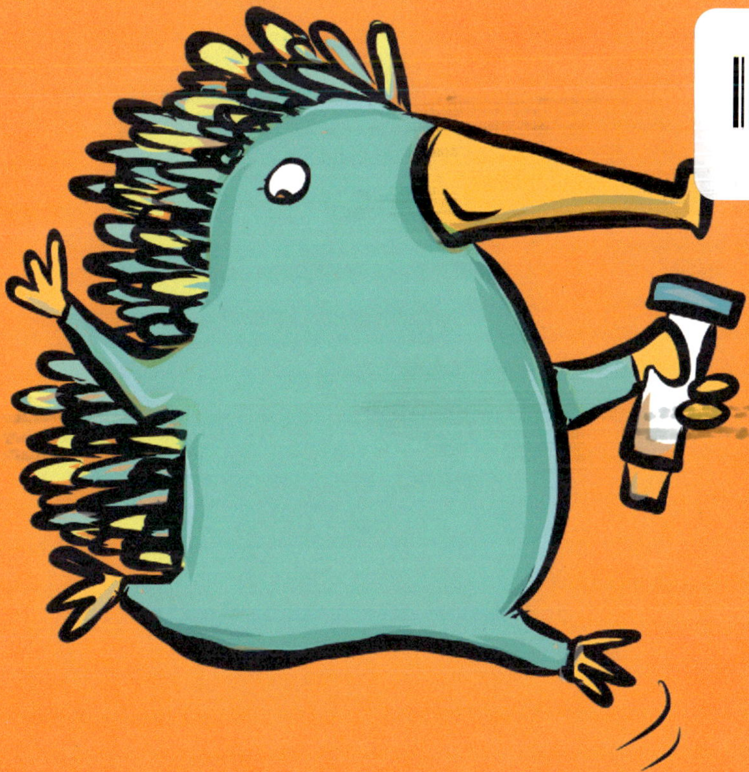

DR. ABRAHAM THOMAS

NEVA THOMAS

light AUSTRALIA

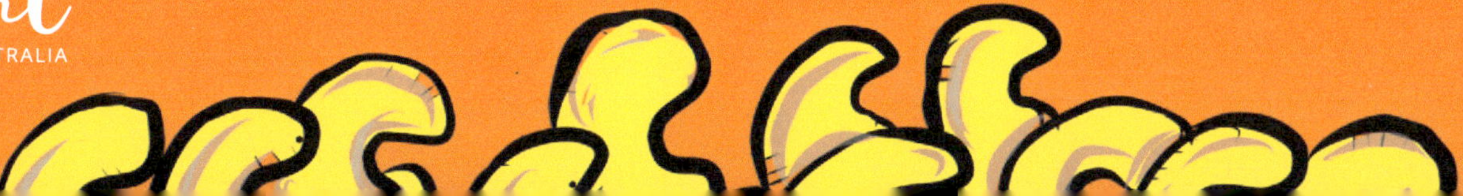

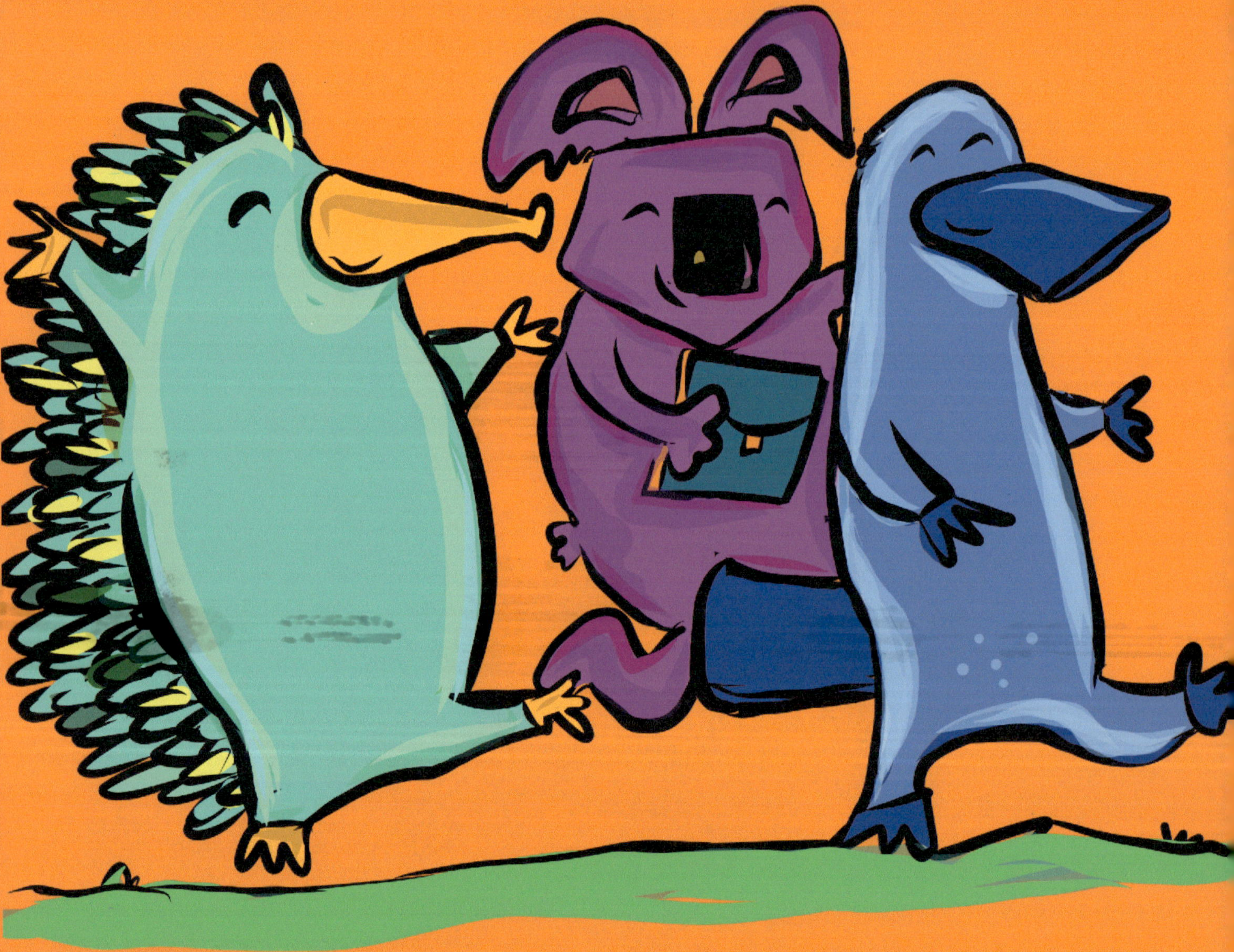

Bobby the echidna was having a picnic with his friends Aiden the platypus & Neva the koala.

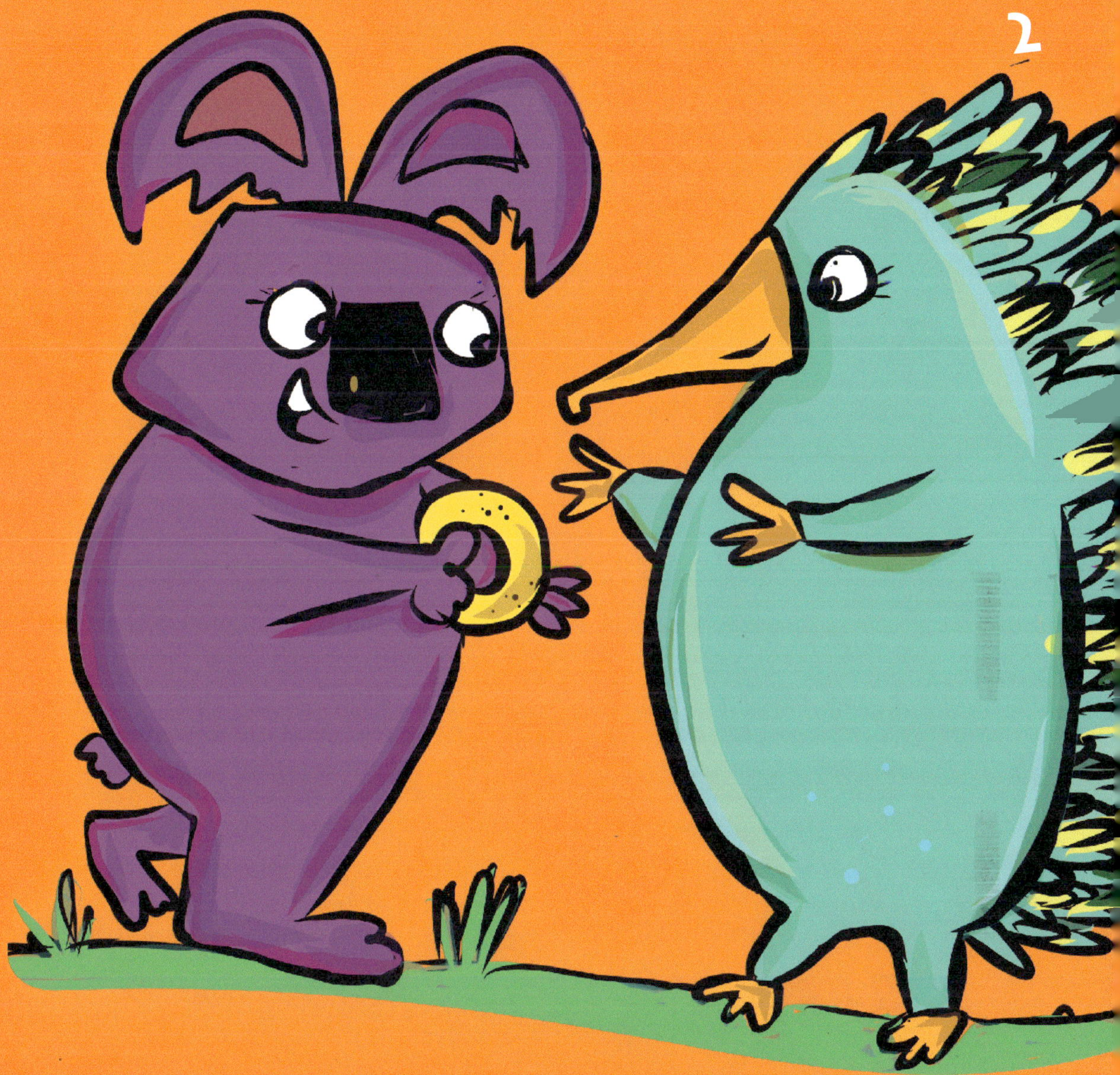

'Try this donut. I got it just for our picnic,' said Neva excitedly. Bobby grabbed the yummy looking donut and started to munch it.

'Waaow ! This tastes yummy,' exclaimed Bobby.

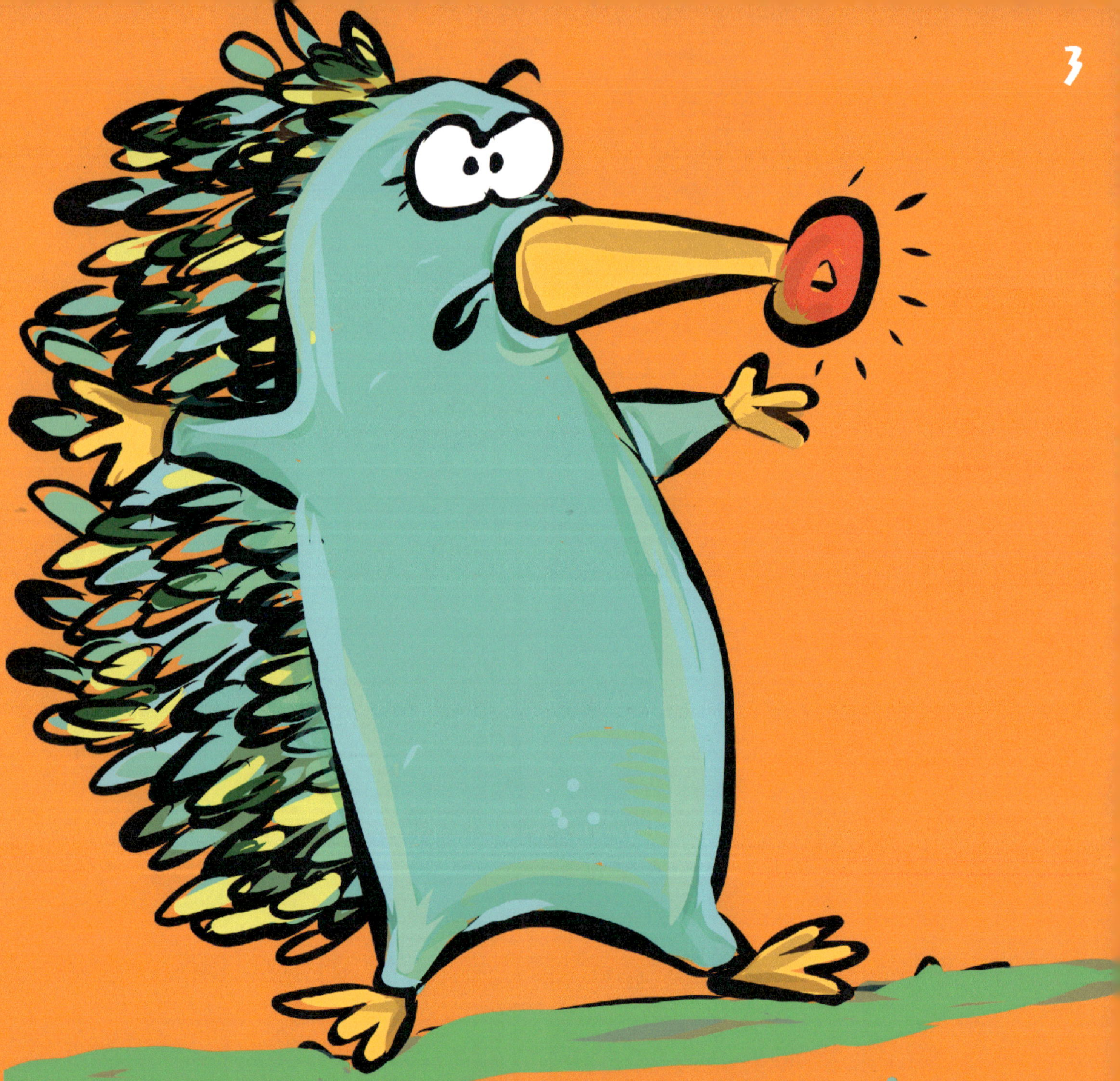

Suddenly Bobby felt that his lips were swelling.

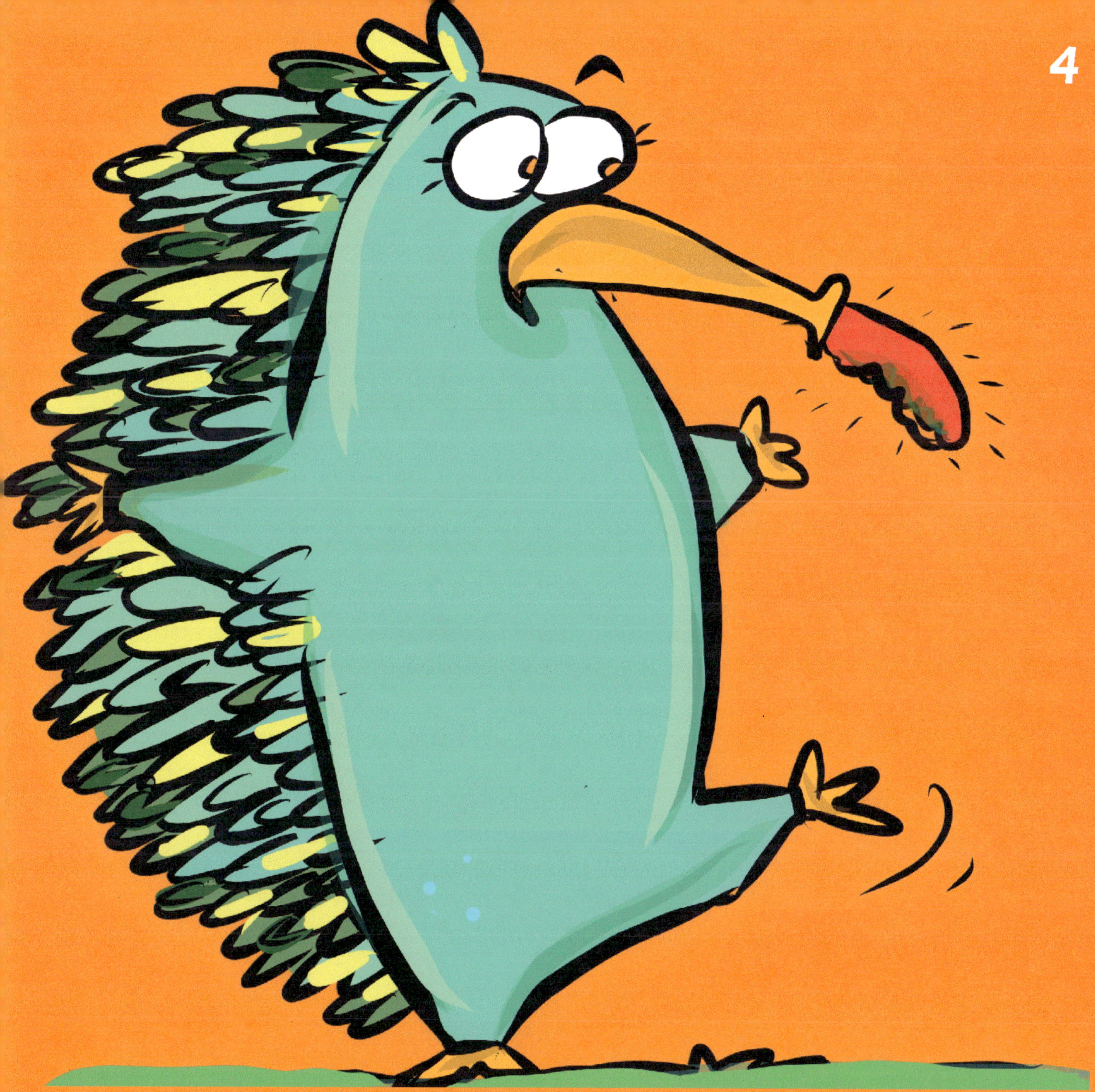

And his tongue!!!

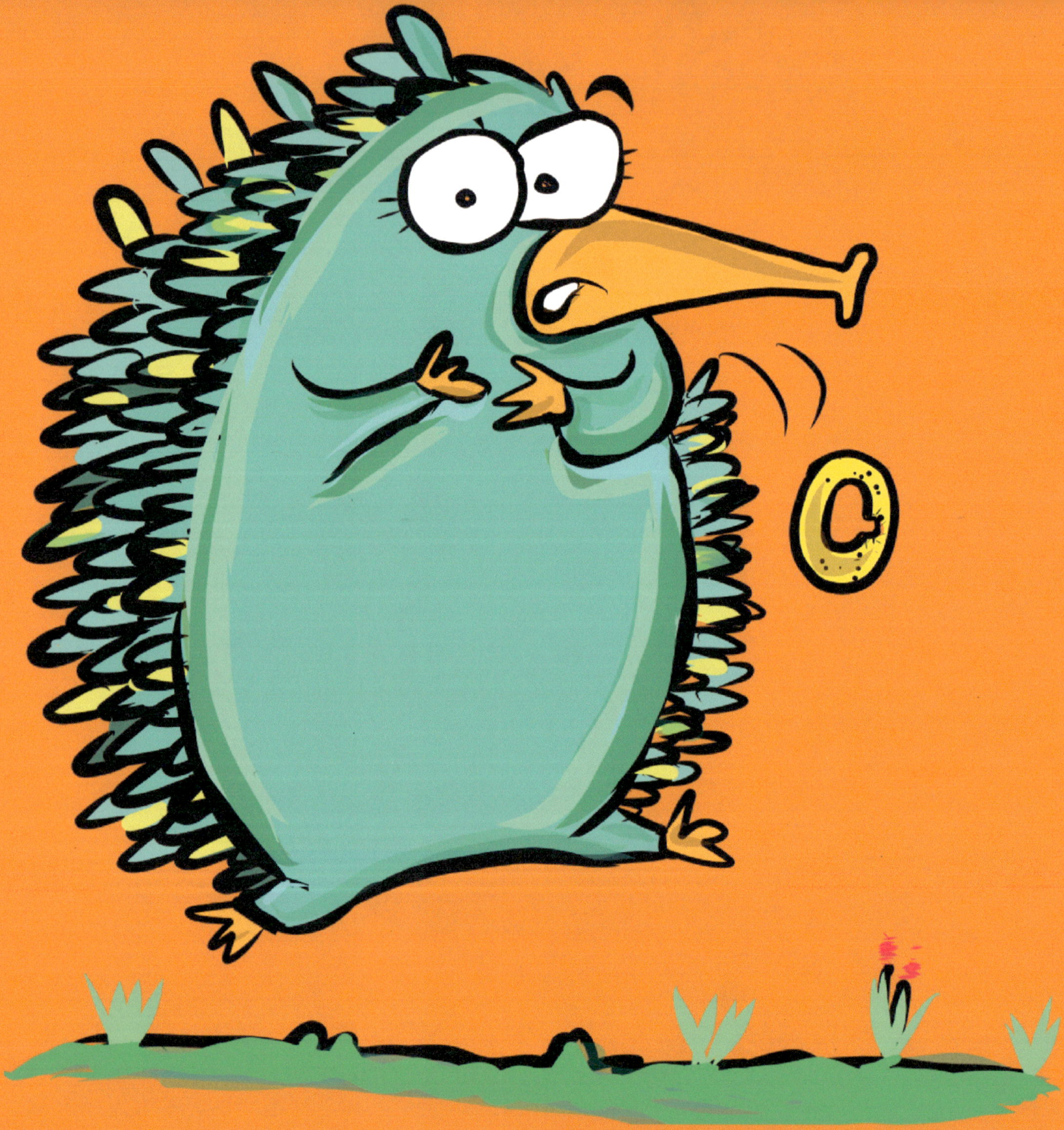

He felt that his throat was swelling too!!

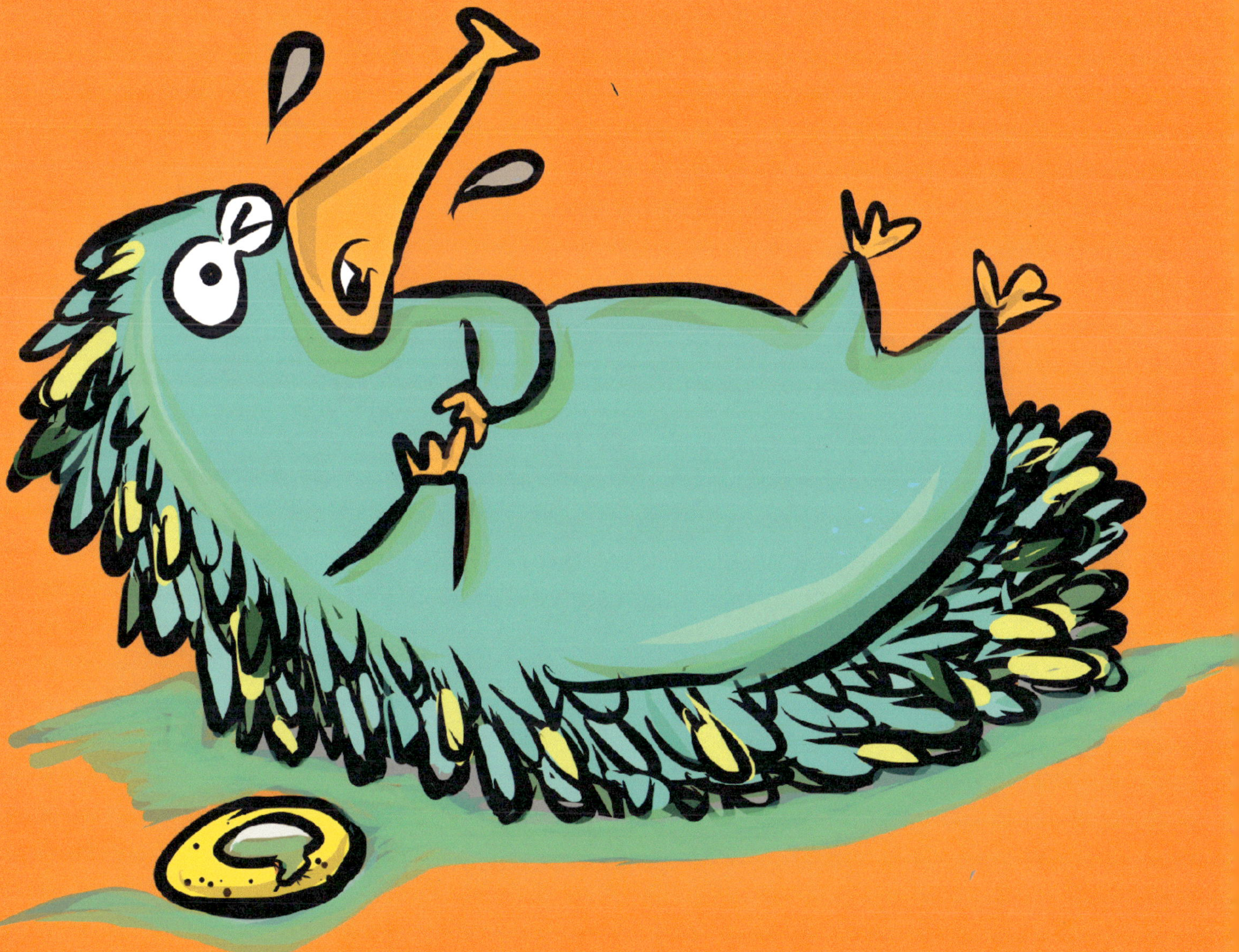

“I can't breathe,' Bobby screamed in panic.

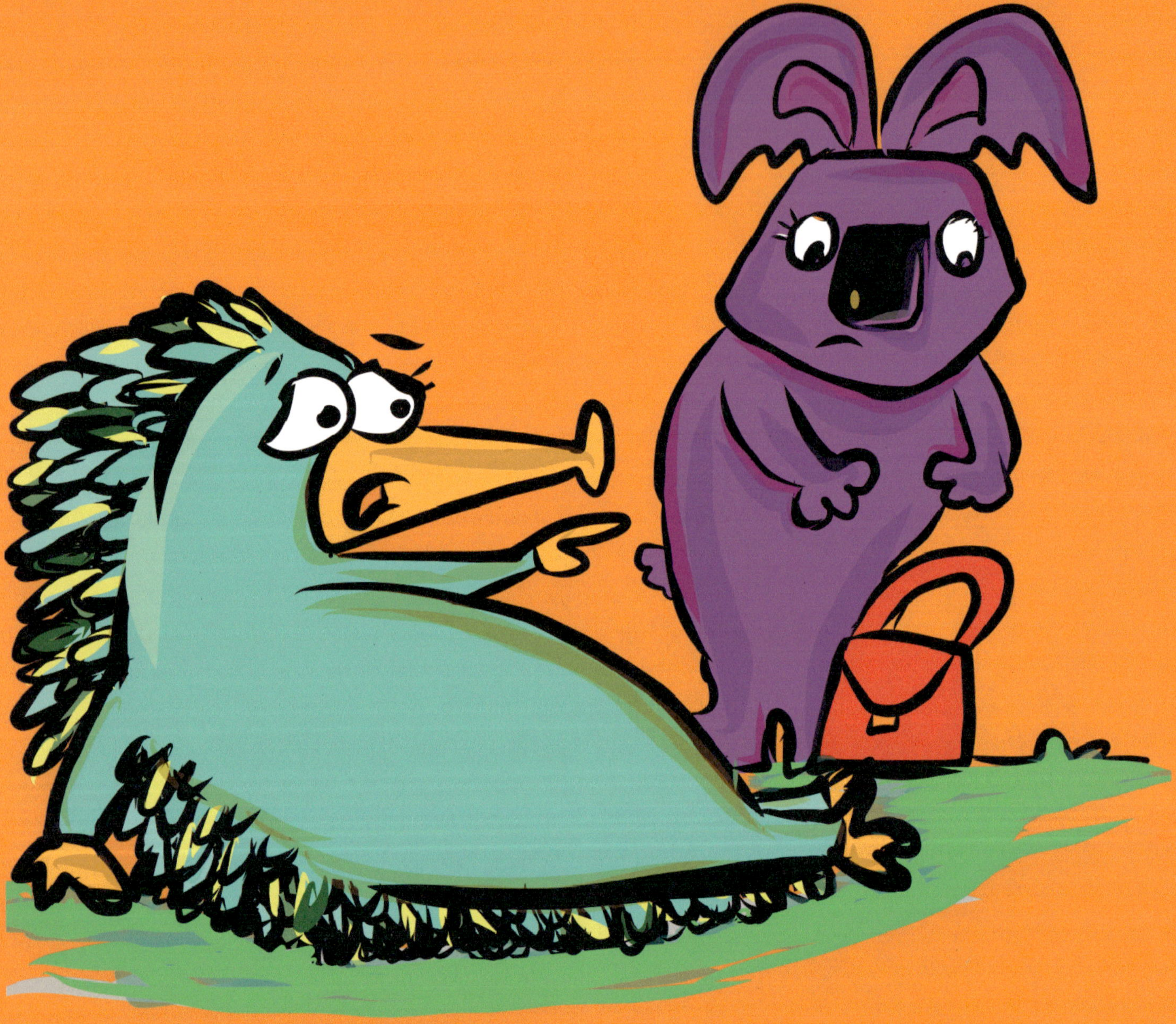

'Can you get me the special medicine pen from my bag quickly Neva 'Bobby screamed.

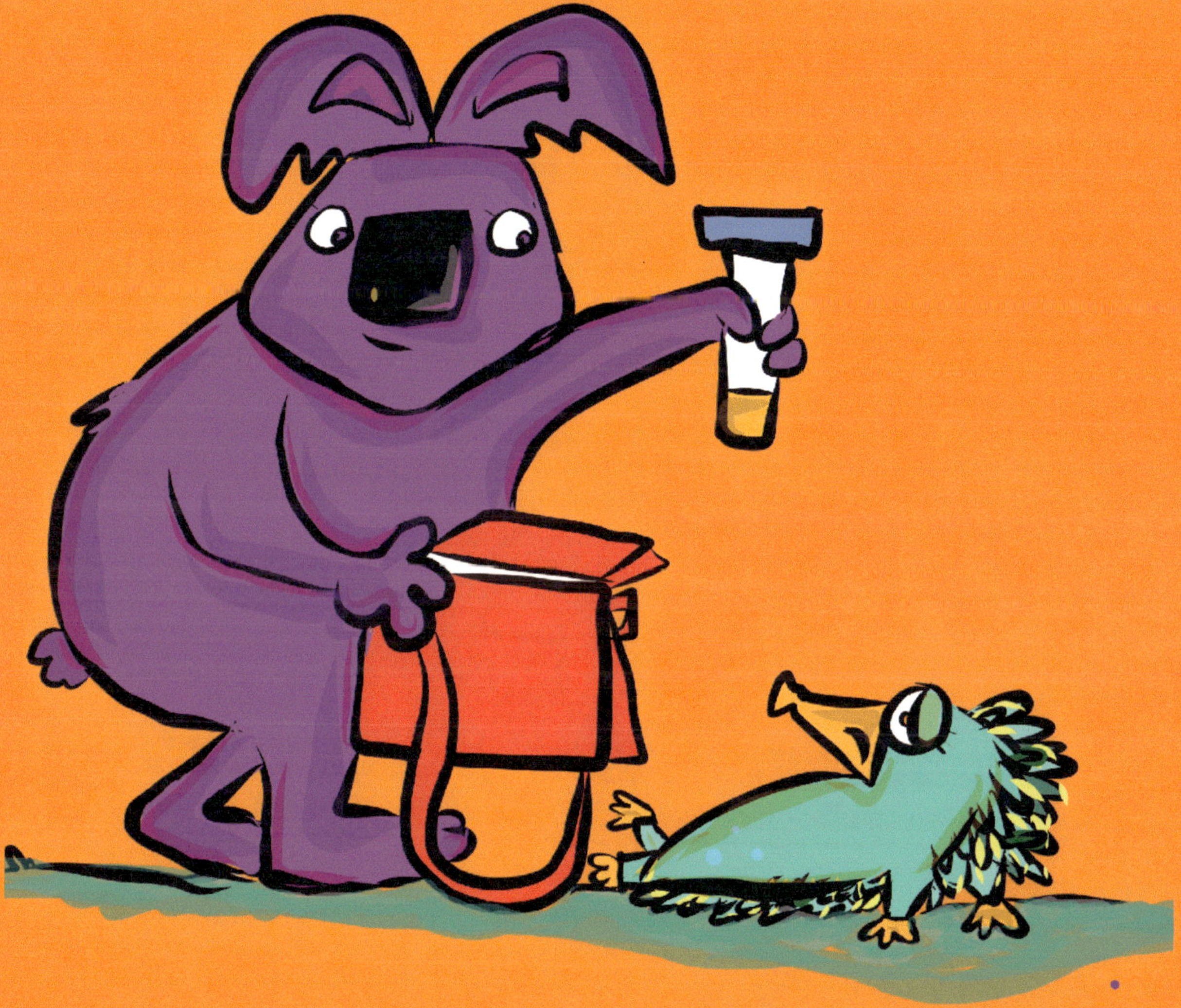

Neva grabbed Bobby's bag and had a good look.
She came across the large orange blue pen kept securely in Bobby's bag and she took it out.
'That is my ADRENALINE PEN which I use in an emergency. I am too sick to give it myself,' said Bobby.

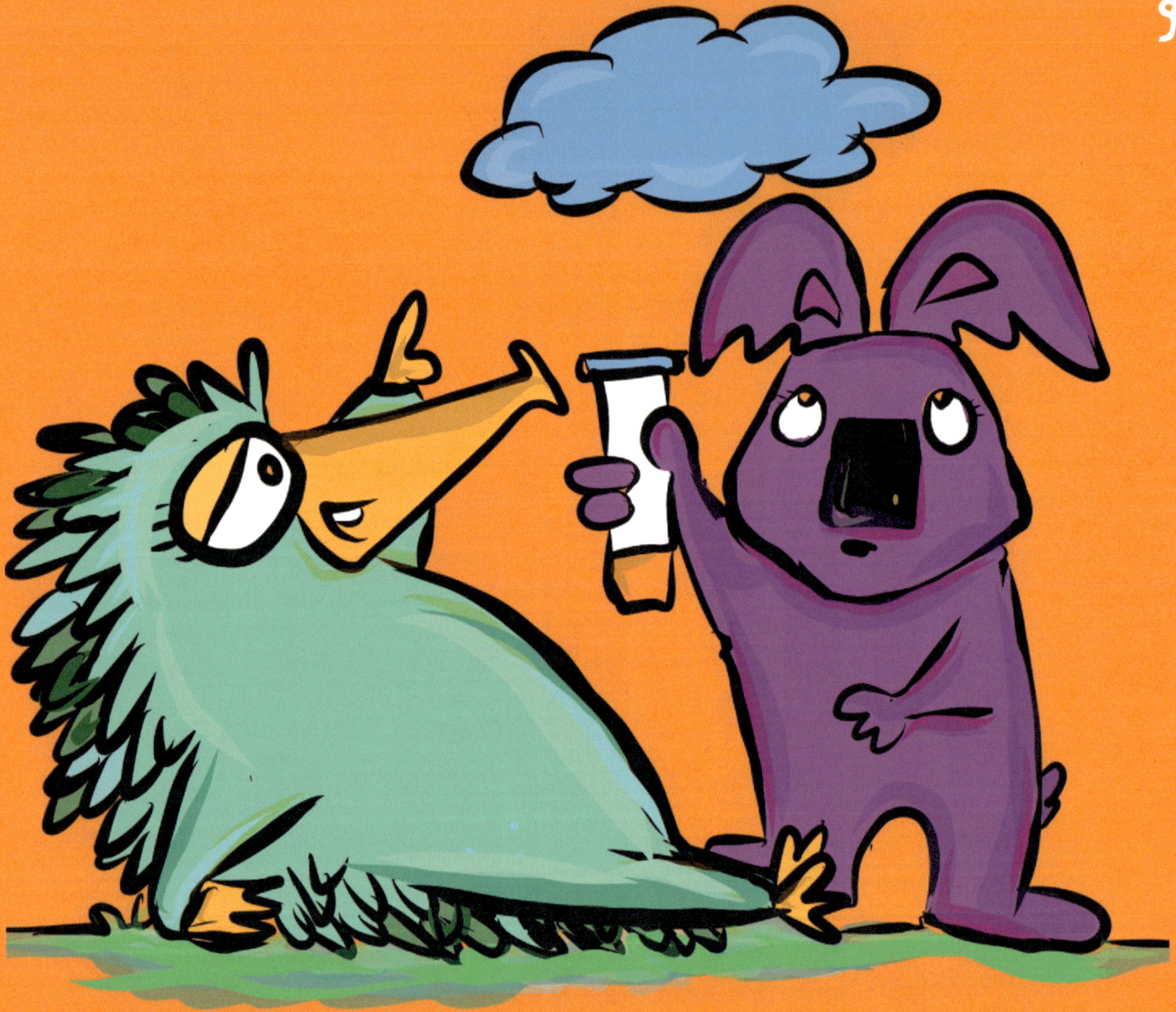

'Neva, please point the blue cap of the pen towards the sky and the orange tip towards my thigh.
Take the blue cap off and jab the orange tip of the pen straight into my thigh quickly', requested Bobby.

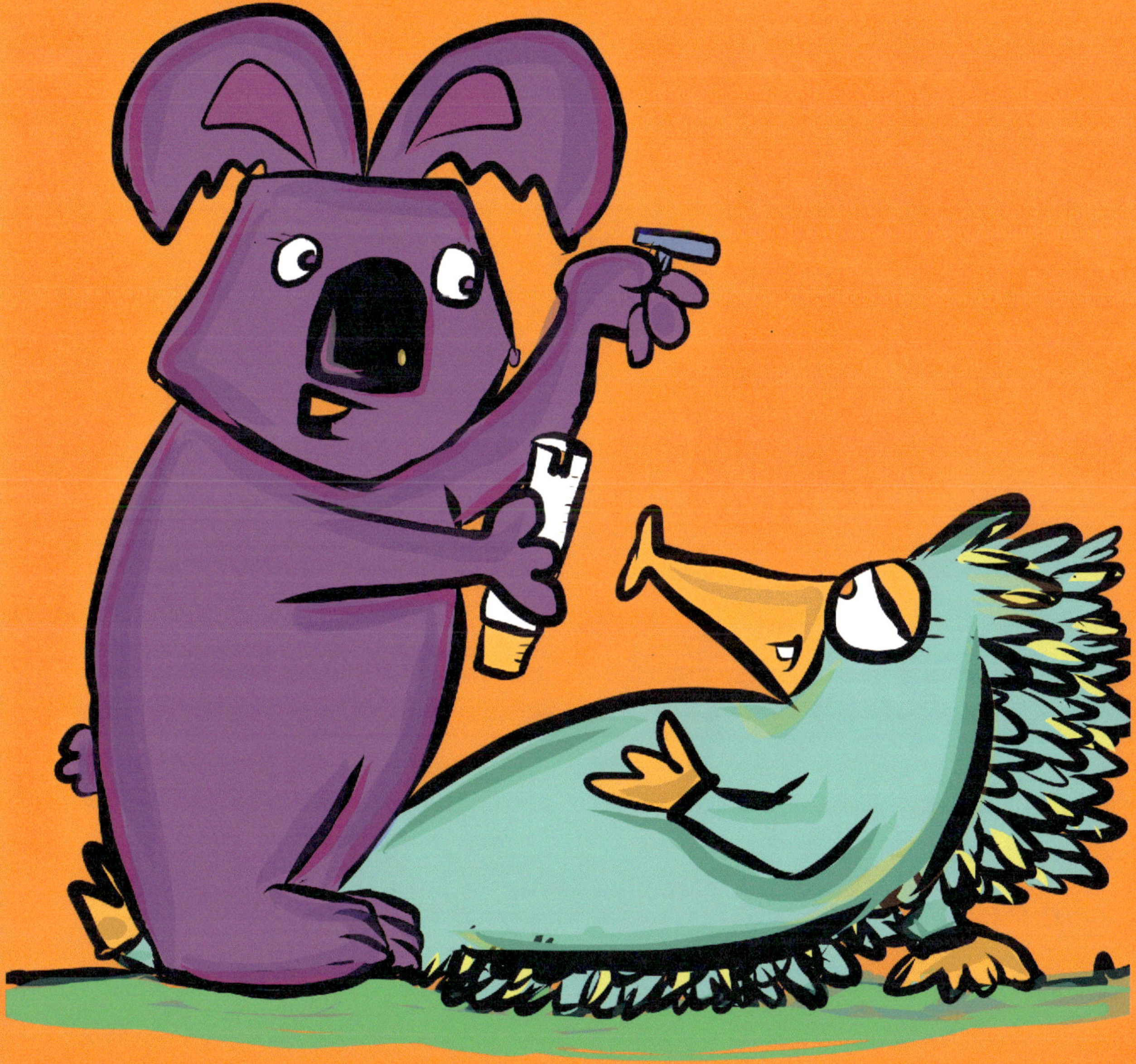

Neva was scared. She said 'Bobby, I have never done this before.'

'Don't worry Neva, I will go through the steps with you,' said Bobby.

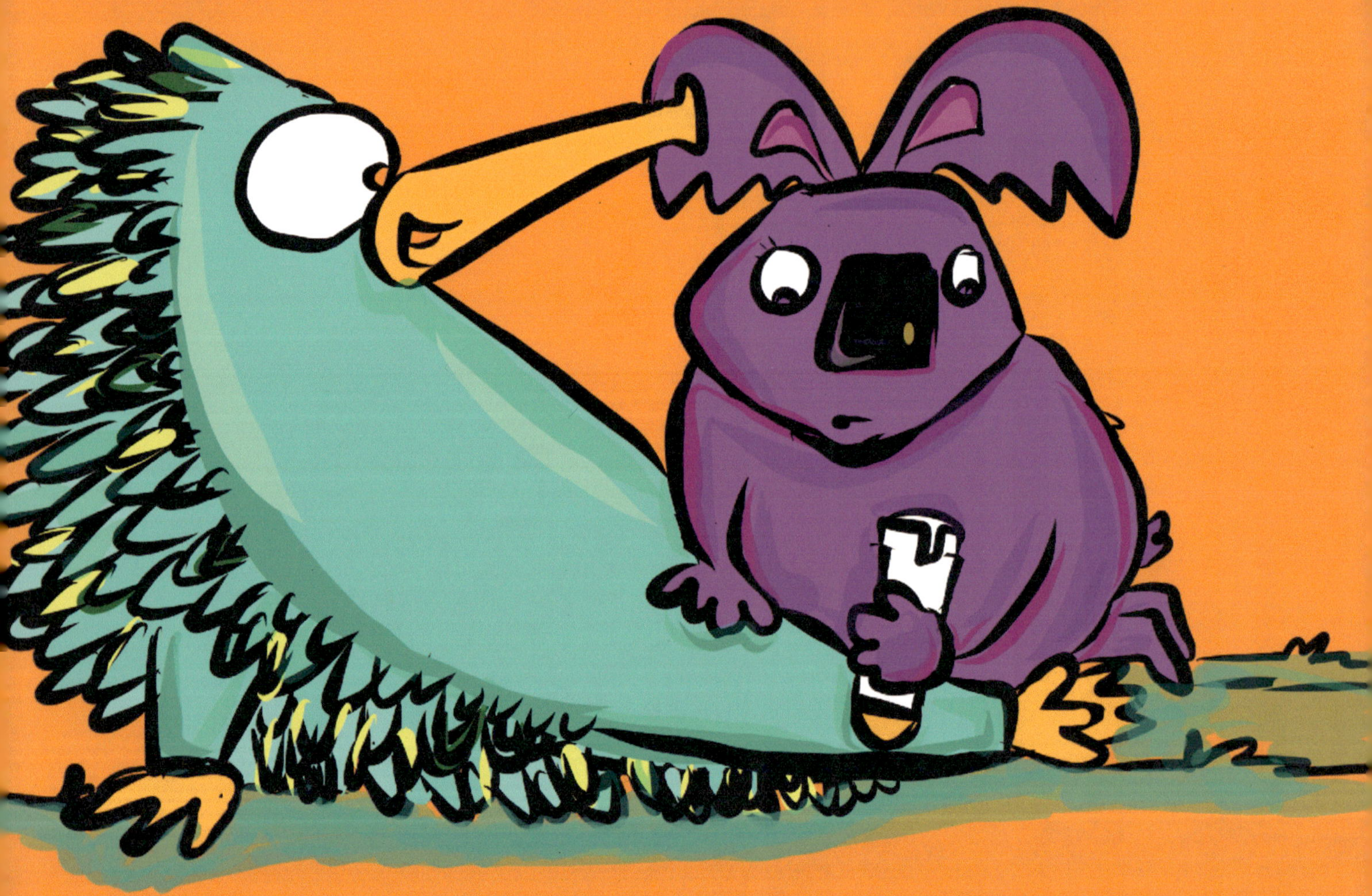

'Please do it as soon as you can,' said Bobby.
Neva took off the blue cap from the top and jabbed the orange tip straight into Bobby's thigh.

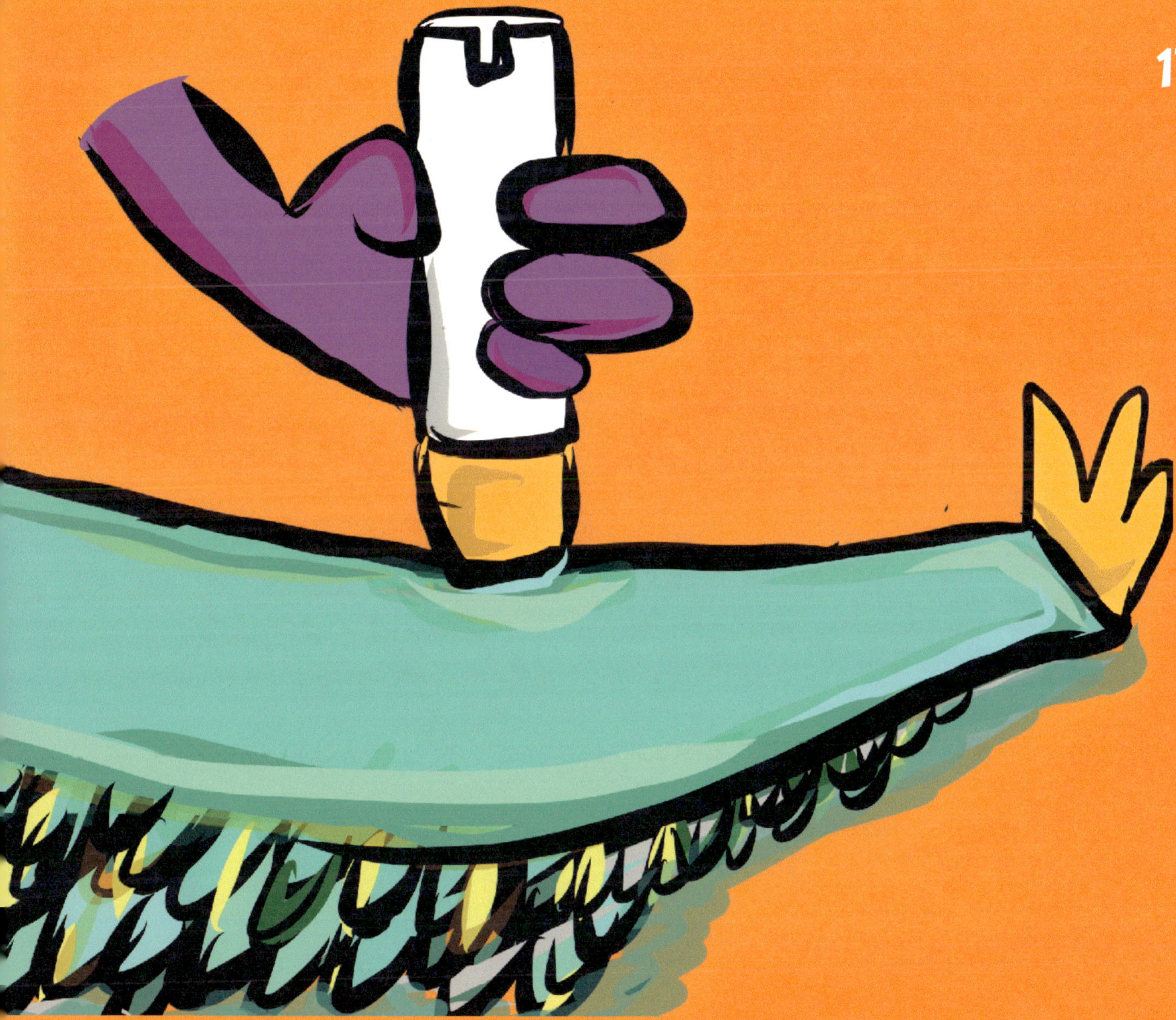

'Well done, hold my Adrenaline Pen for 10 seconds Neva,' said Bobby

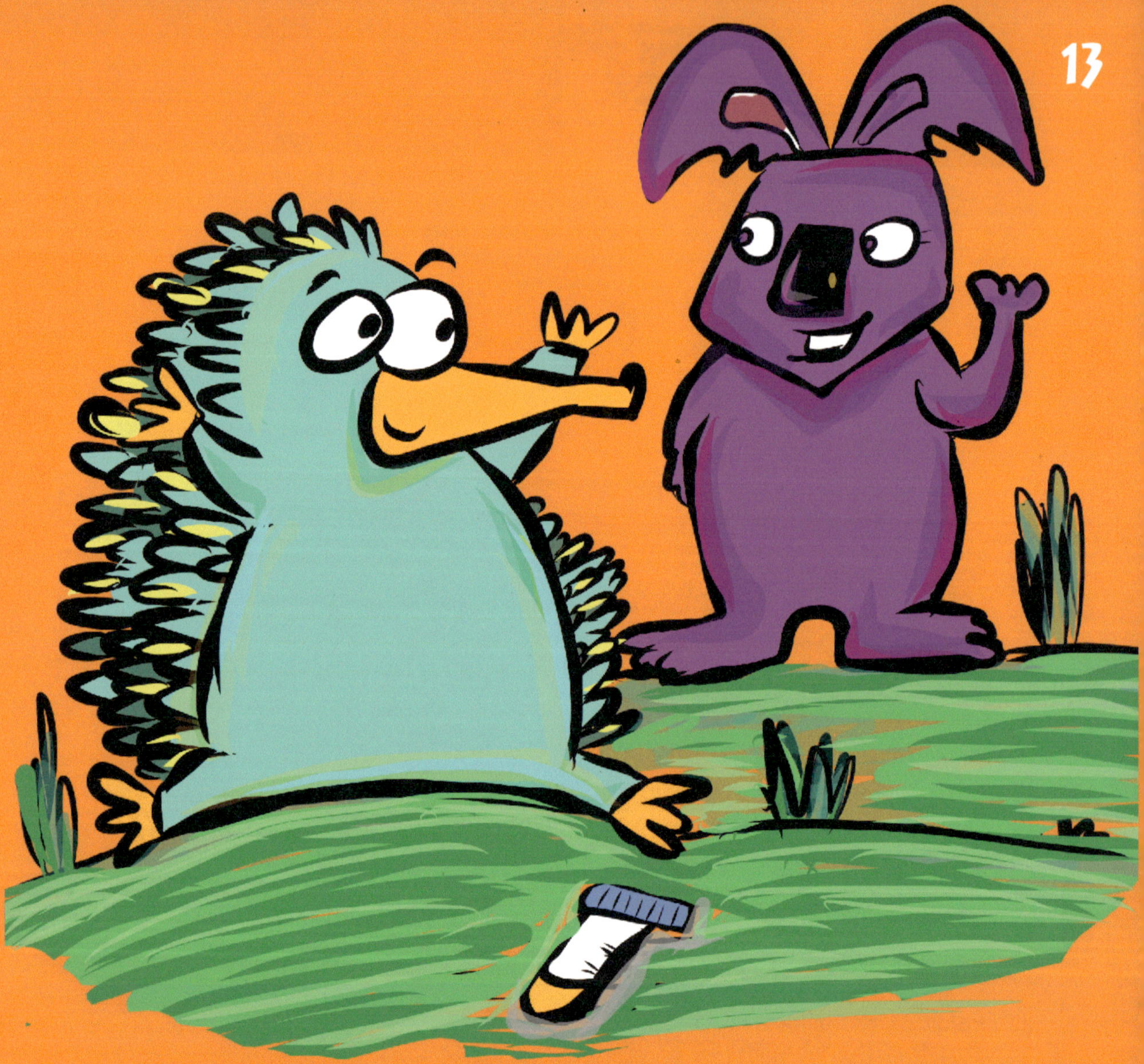

In a few minutes ...
'I feel much better now. I can breathe better. My lip and tongue swelling has gone down. Thank you Neva,' Bobby smiled in relief.

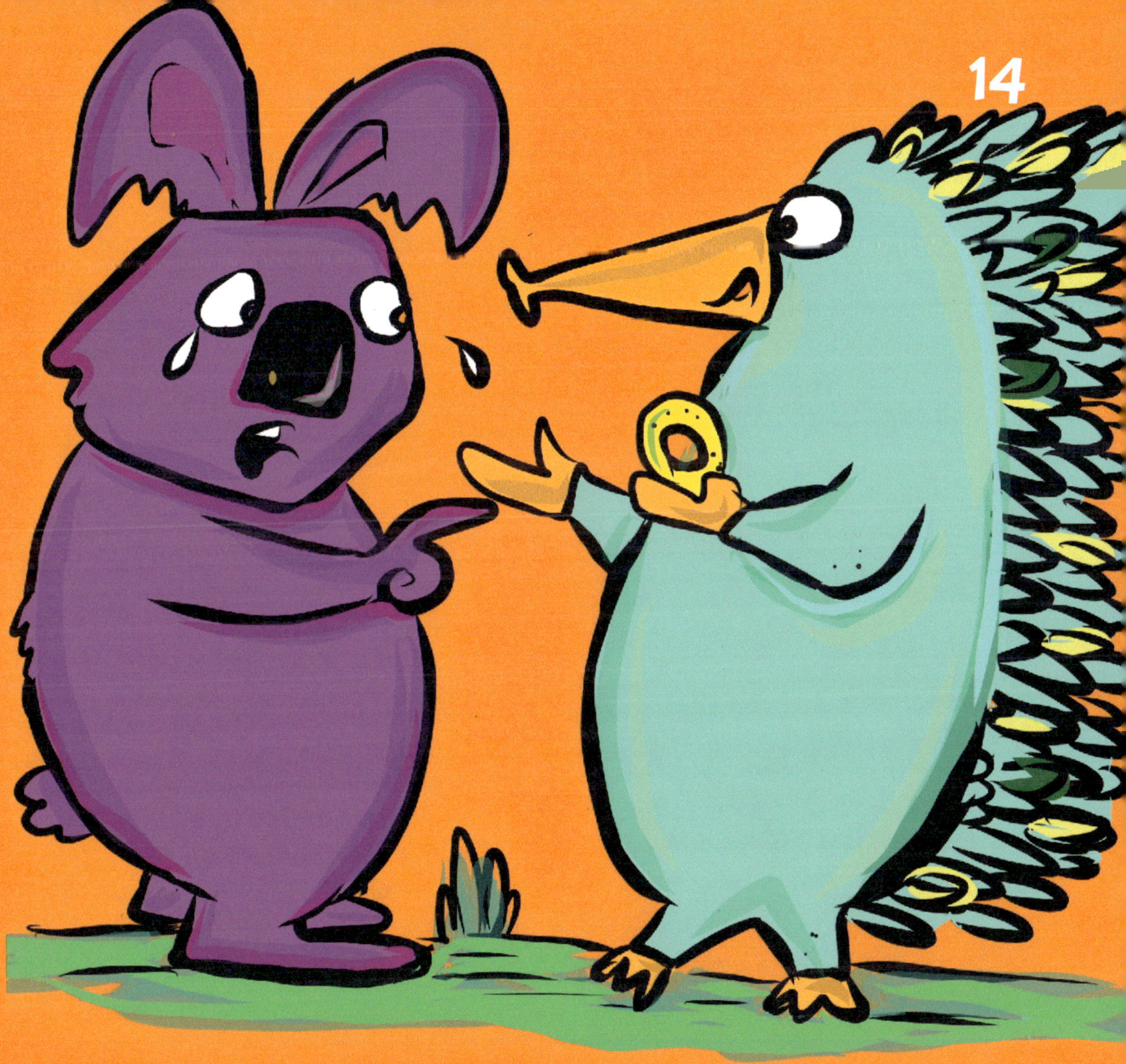

Neva was in a state of shock with all what has happened around her.

She asked Bobby,' What exactly happened Bobby?'

'I had a BAD FOOD ALLERGIC REACTION to nuts in the donut you gave me Neva!' said Bobby.

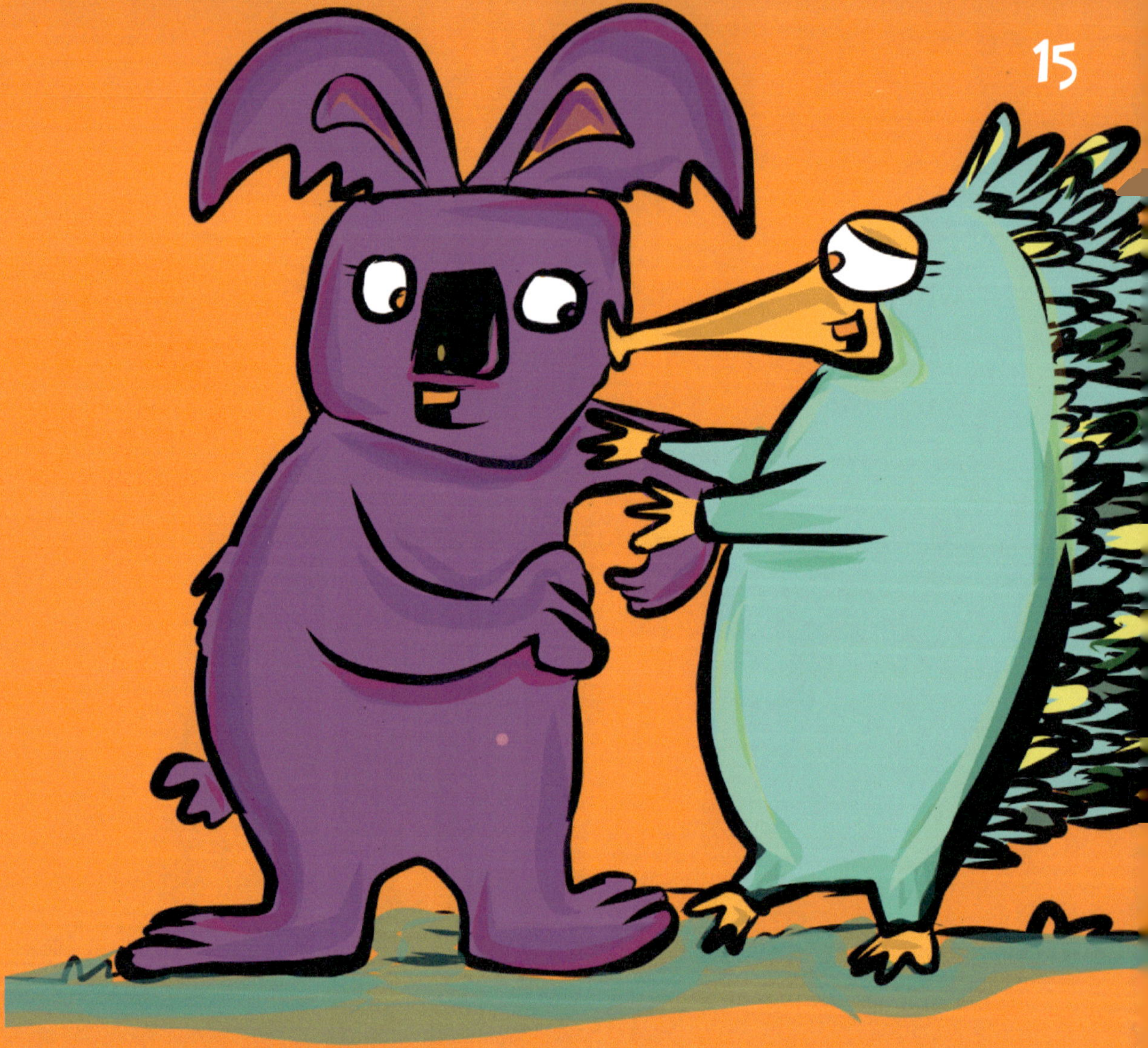

'I am so sorry Bobby! I didn't know that you have such a bad FOOD ALLERGY,' cried Neva.

'It is not your fault Neva. I should have checked it with you in the first place.

I have ANAPHYLAXIS to nuts,' explained Bobby.

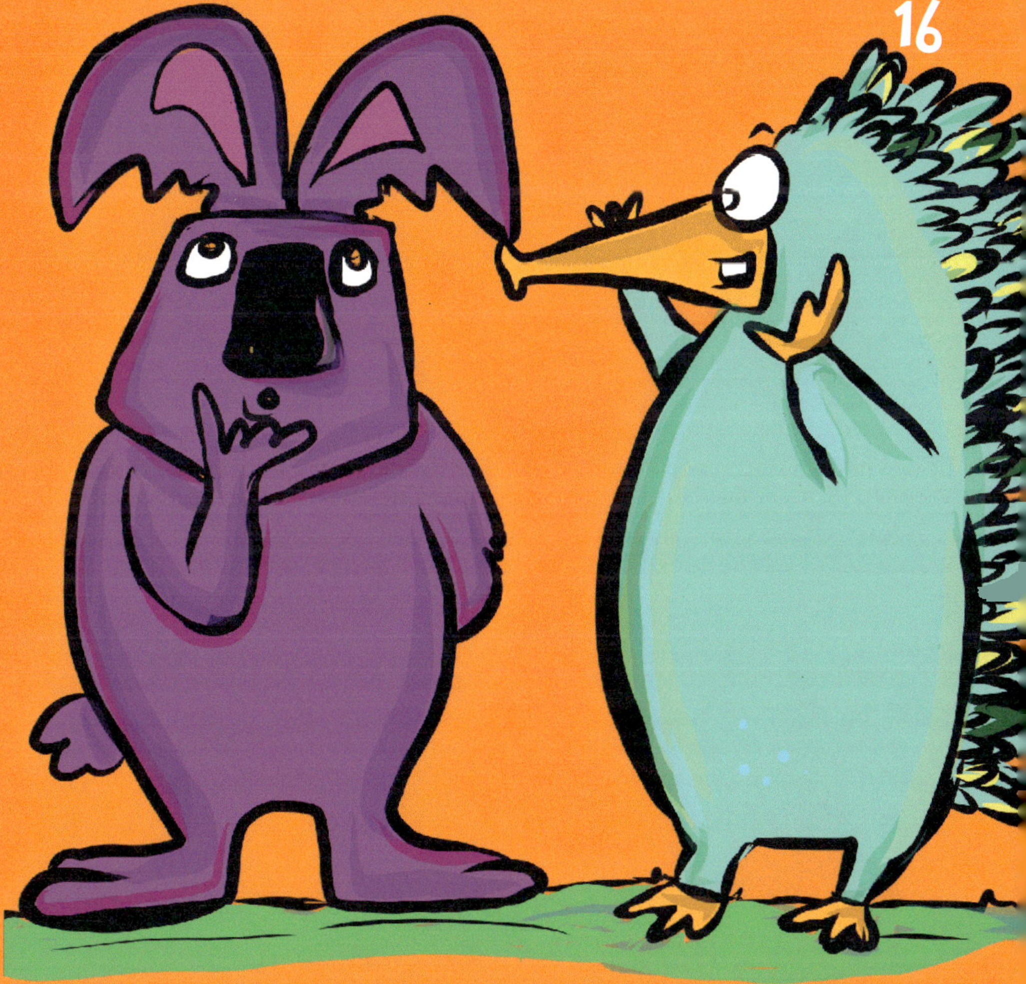

'ANAPHYLAXIS?? What is it?' asked Neva confused.
'It is a VERY BAD ALLERGIC REACTION to certain food stuffs. For me it is NUTS. It can cause my tongue and lips to swell up and my throat can close up too. I will have big trouble breathing if this happens.' explained Bobby.

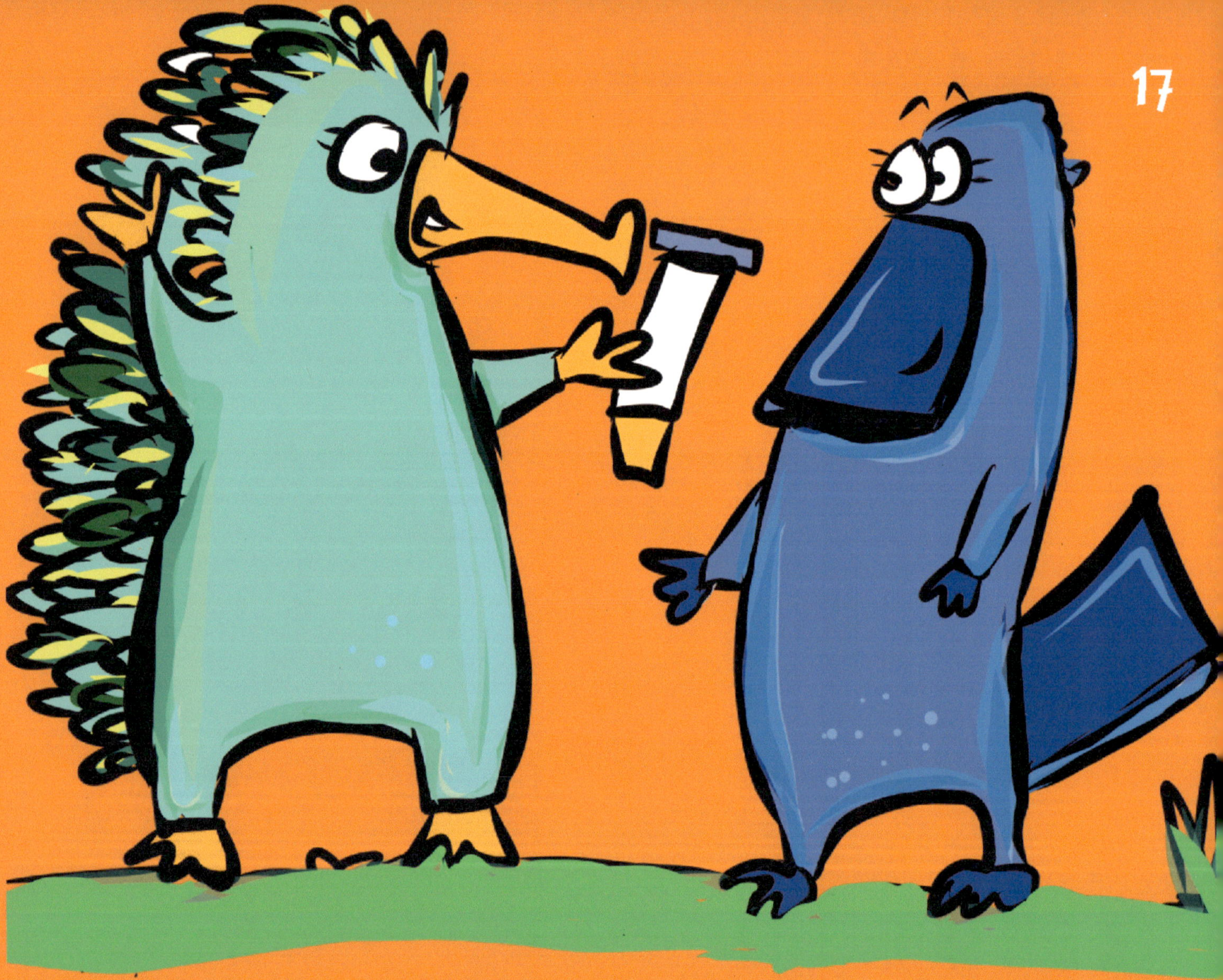

'So I carry this special medicine called ADRENALINE, which I take straight away. If I don't take the medicine in this pen immediately, I will get really sick and end up in Hospital.' said Bobby.

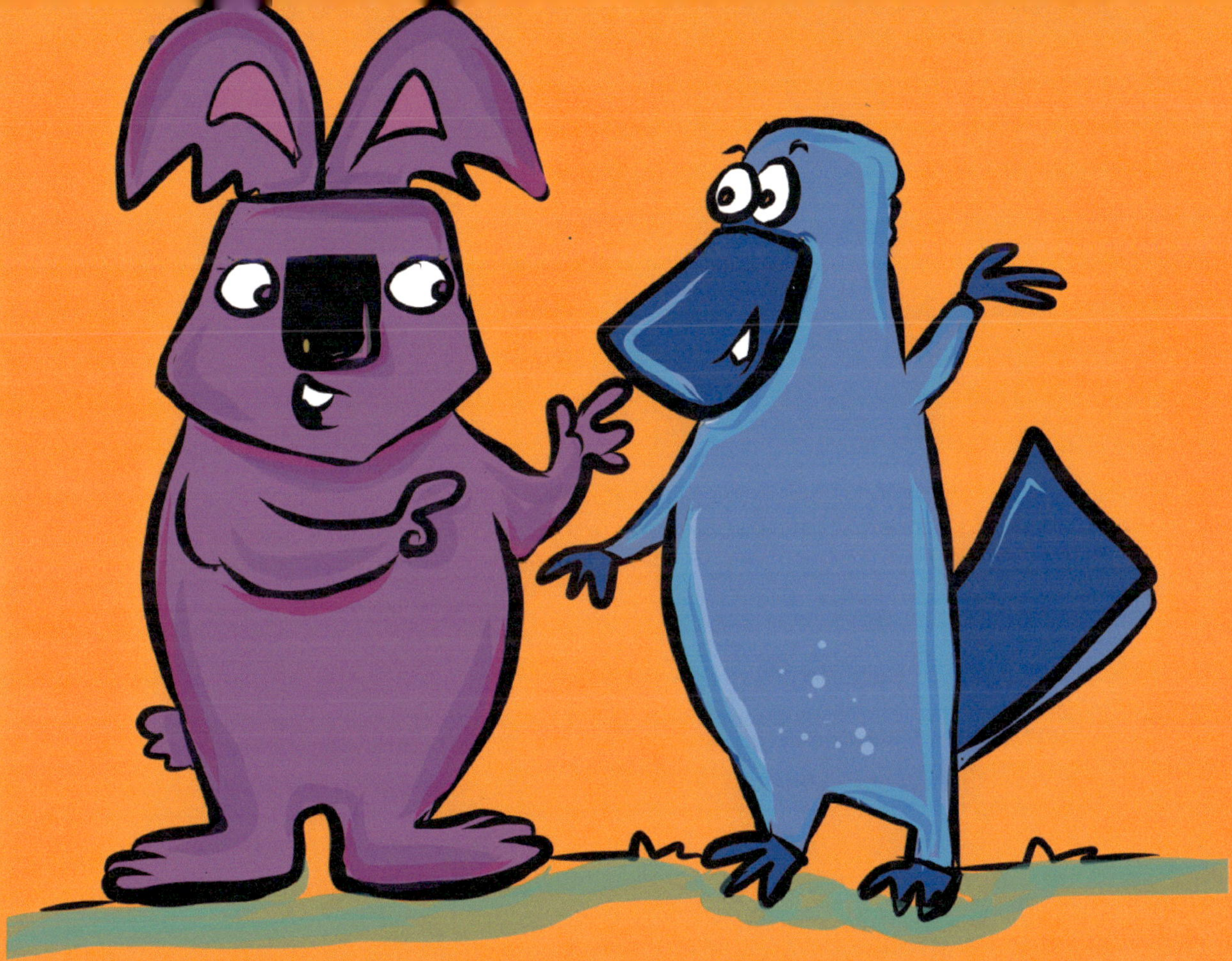

'My sister has allergy to nuts. She will break into a rash if she eats anything with nuts in it. She takes a special liquid medicine called ANTI HISTAMINES, and she gets better straightaway.' said Neva.

'That is a MILD FOOD ALLERGY Neva. But Bobby has a very severe allergy to nuts that requires this special needle ADRENALINE.' chipped in Aiden.

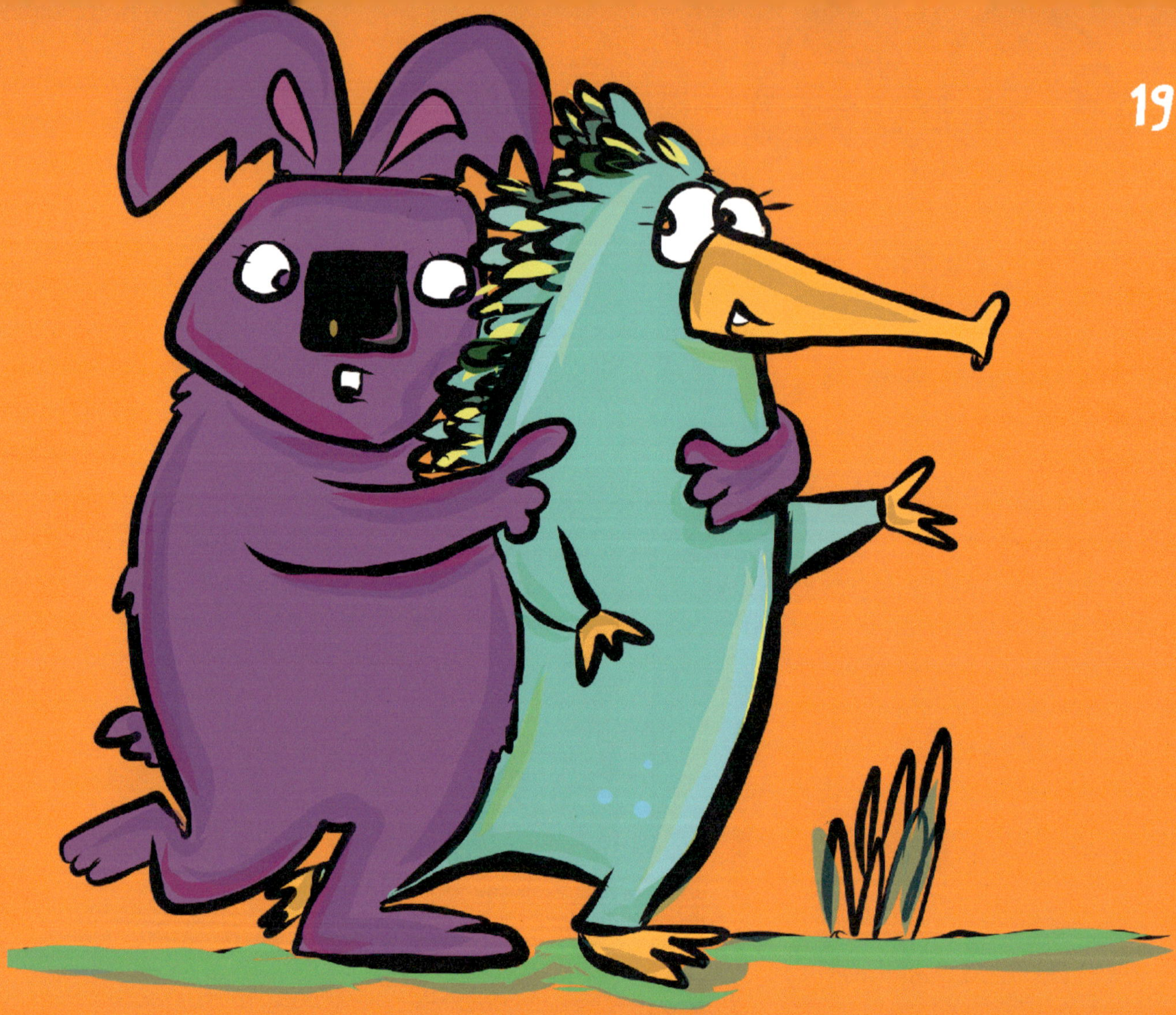

'How did you pick up your food allergy Bobby?' asked Neva.

'I had a similar bad reaction to nuts last year where I ended up in Hospital. They had to give me ADRENALINE at the Hospital.' said Bobby.

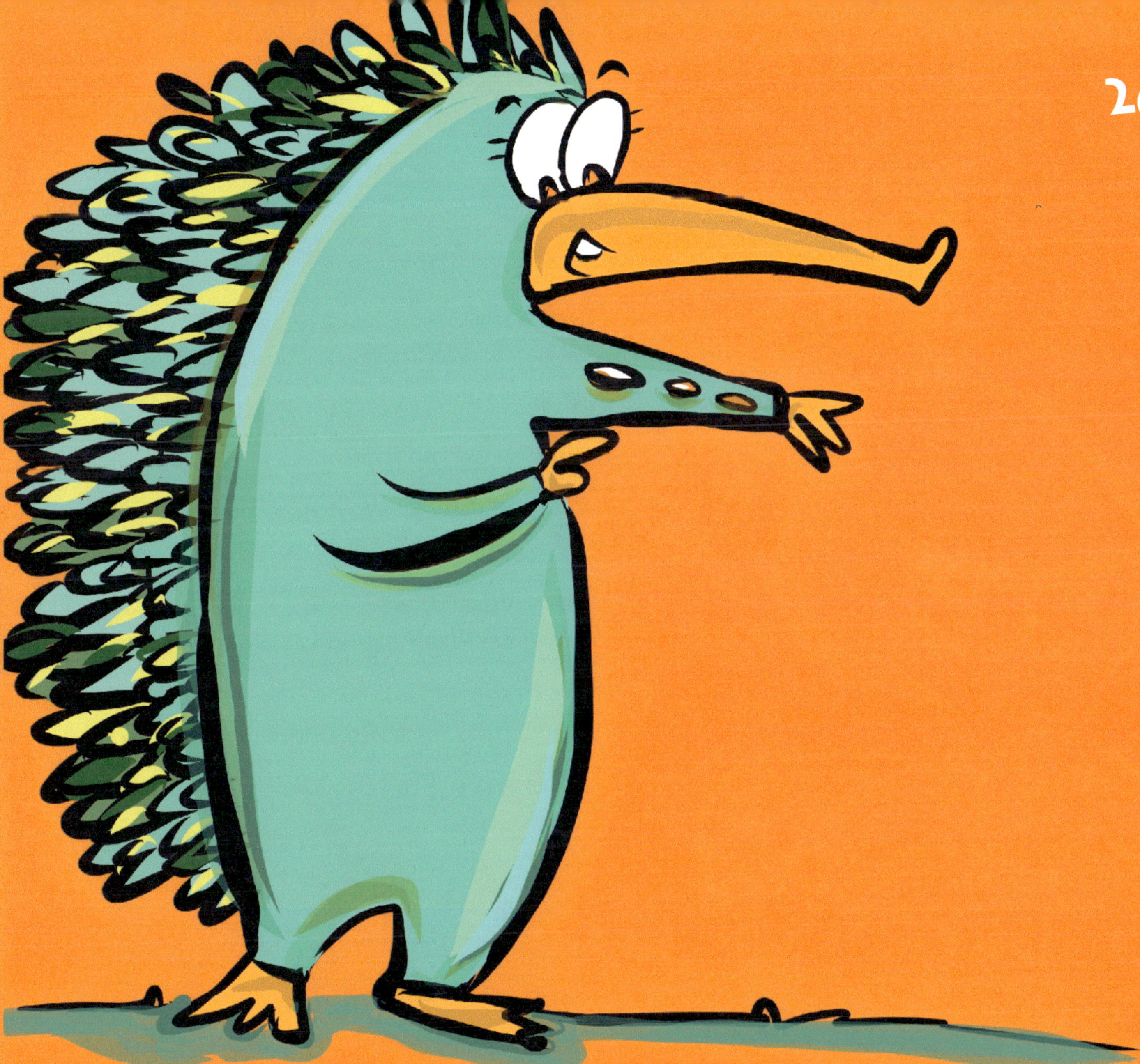

'They later did a special test called the SKIN PRICK TEST, where they injected a few stuffs into my skin.' continued Bobby.

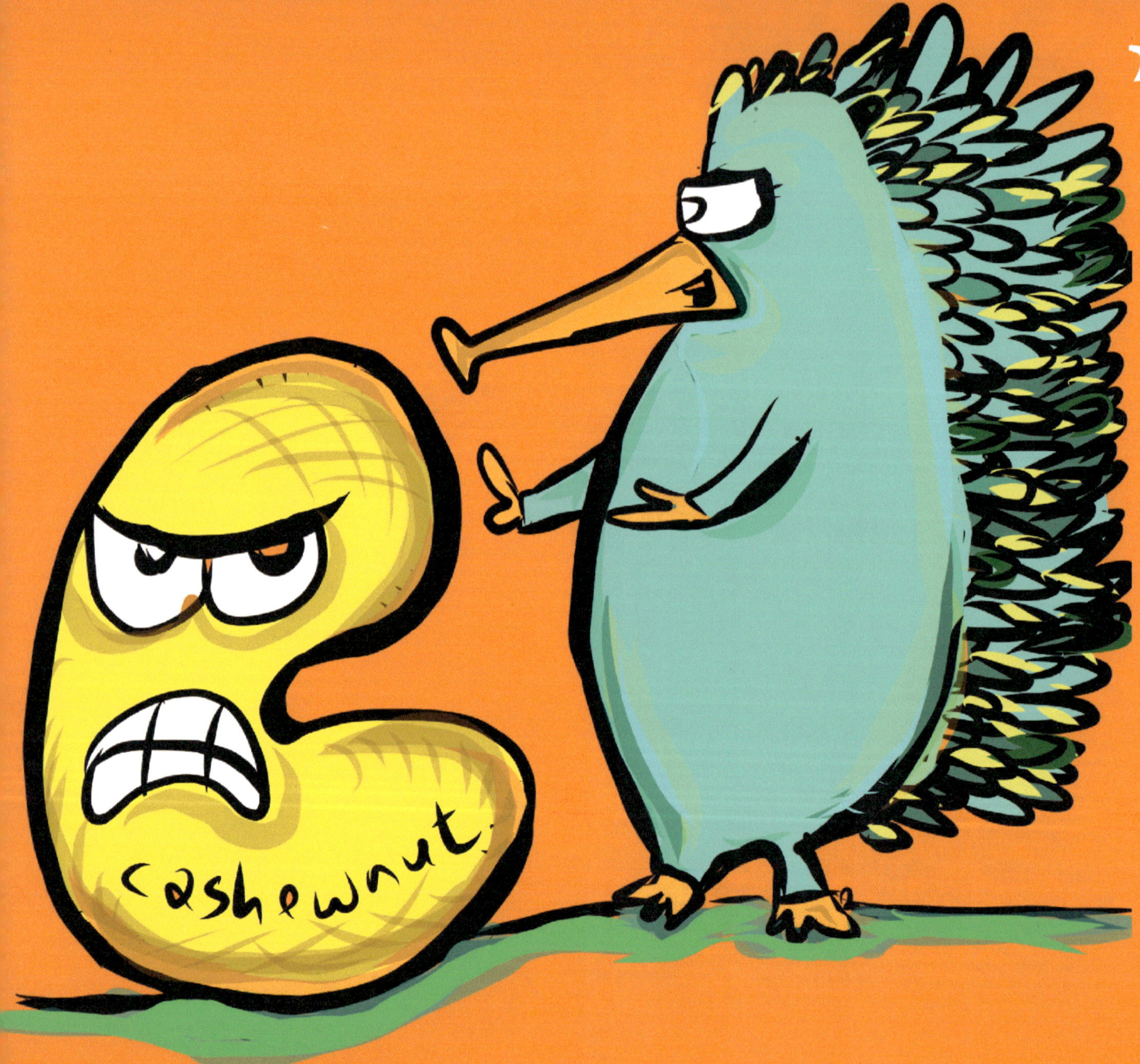

'They found out that I have bad allergy to cashew nuts.' said Bobby.

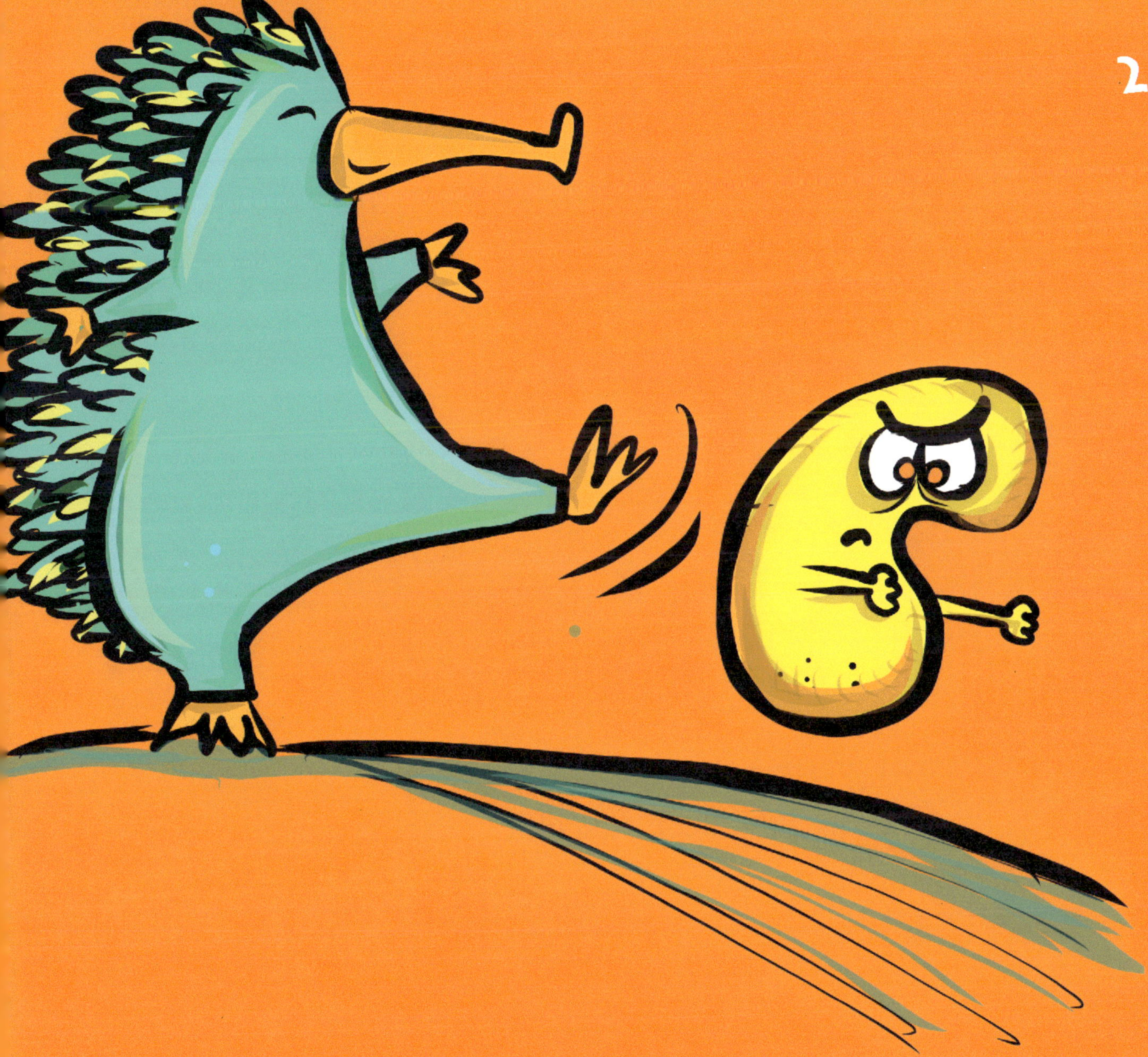

'How did you get over it?' asked Neva curiously.
'I try to avoid taking any foodstuffs with cashew nut in them.' replied Bobby.

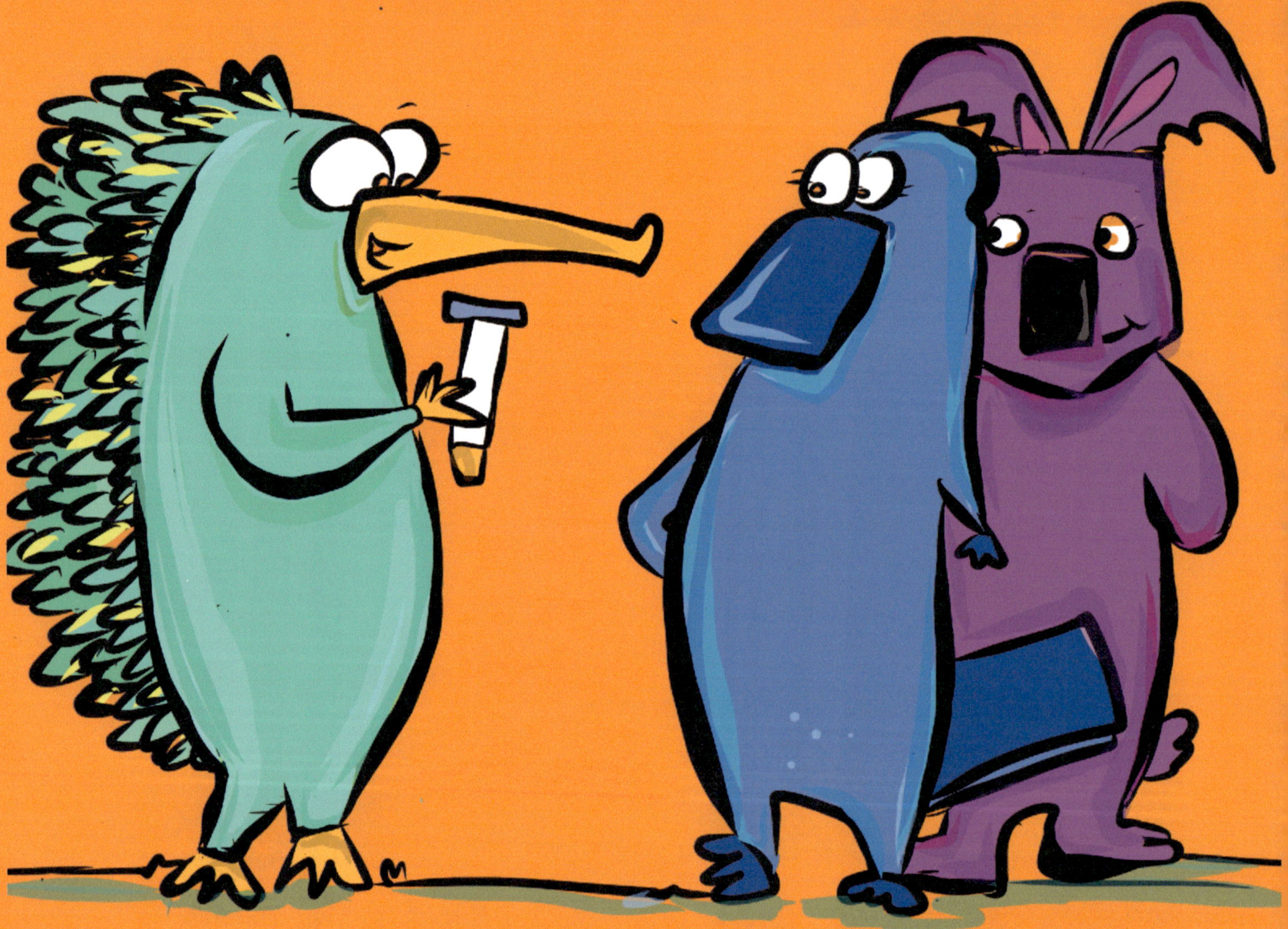

'If I accidentally take anything with cashew nuts and get a bad allergic reaction, I carry this special medicine called ADRENALINE all the time to help me out.' quipped Bobby.

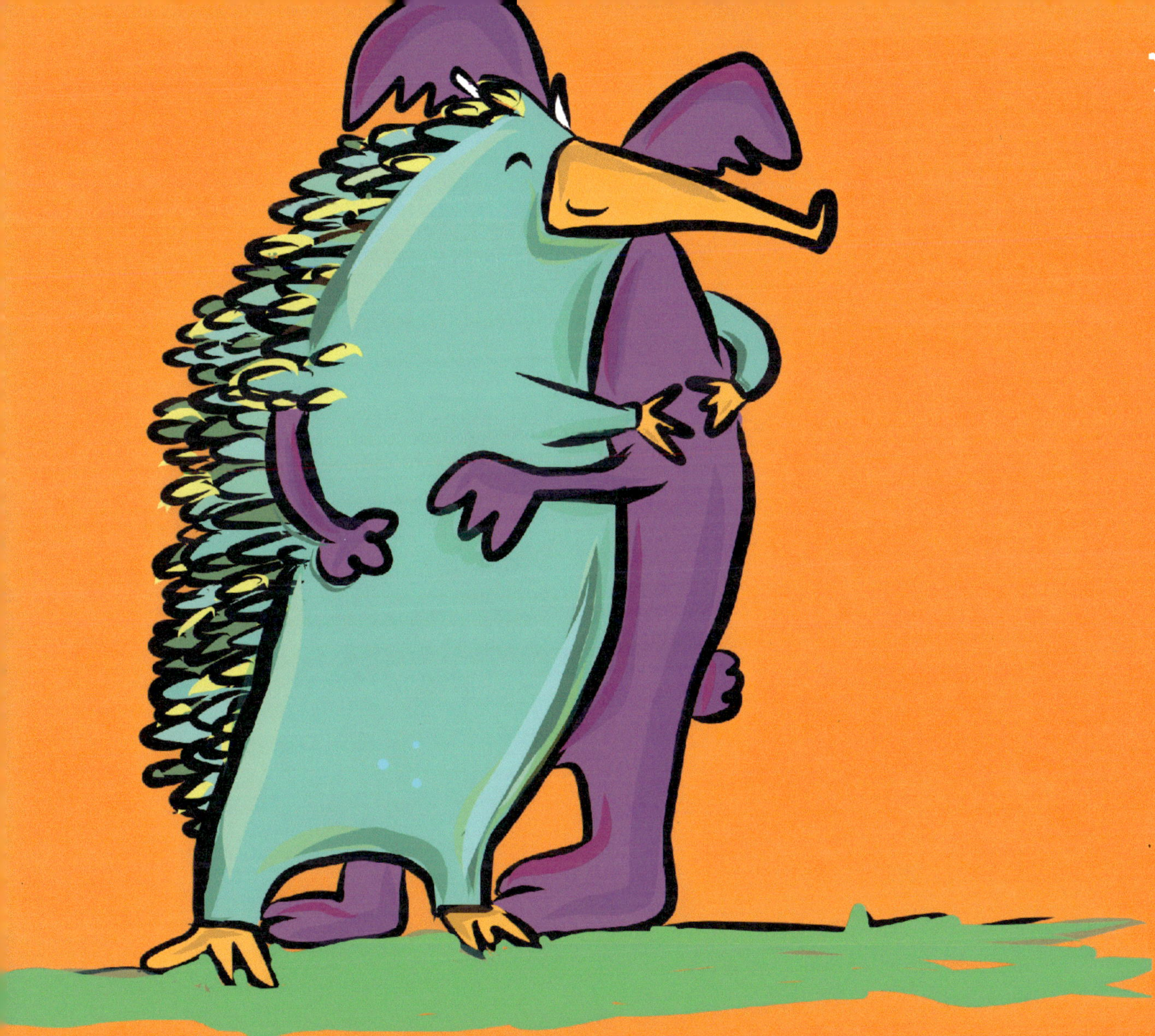

Bobby hugged Neva and said, 'Don't worry Neva, you saved my life today.'

Everyone cheered Neva 'Hurray! Neva is a star, she saved Bobby's life!'

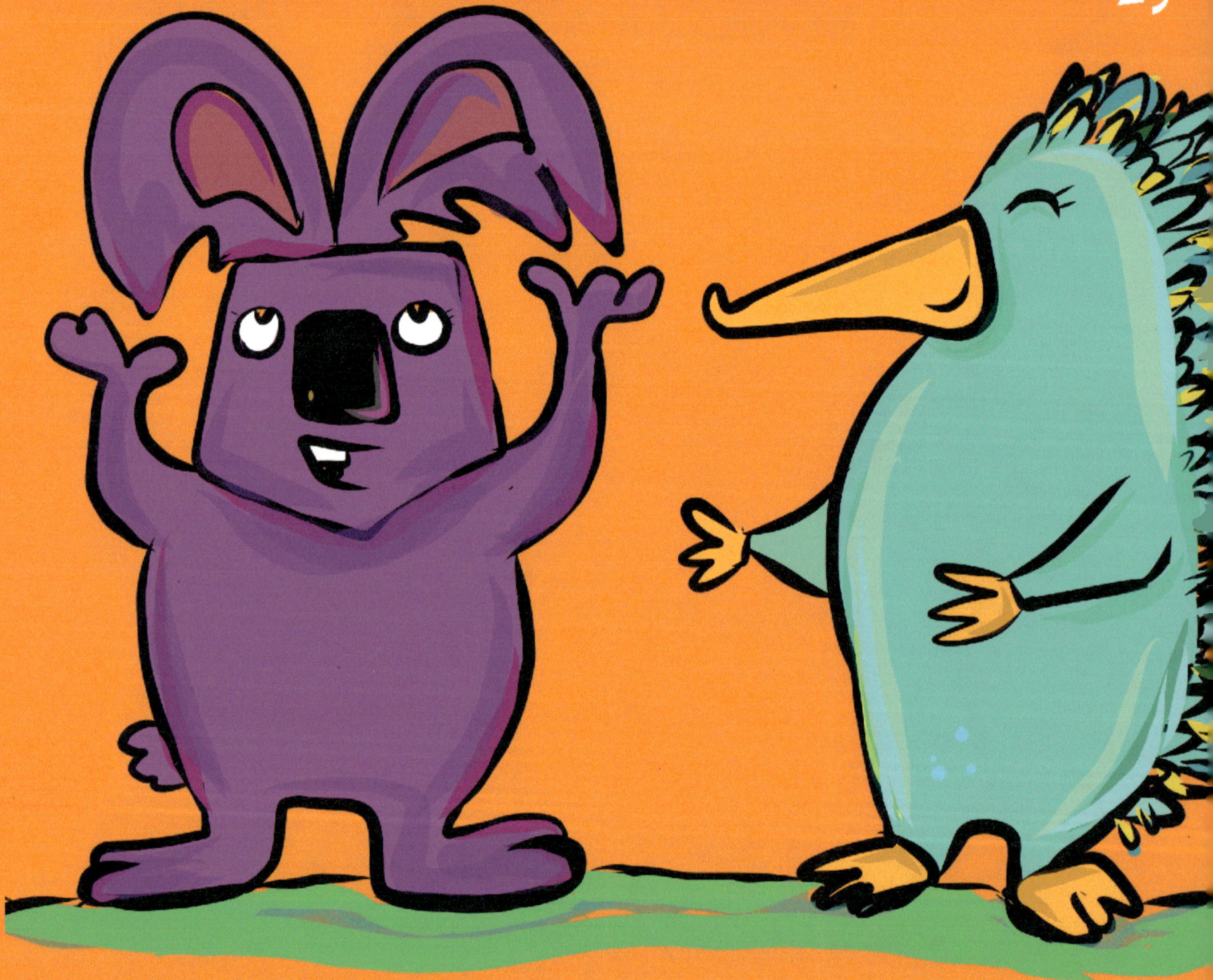

'Now I feel better. I was so sad to make you sick today with my donut.' said Neva.

Neva was feeling less guilty now with all that happened that day.

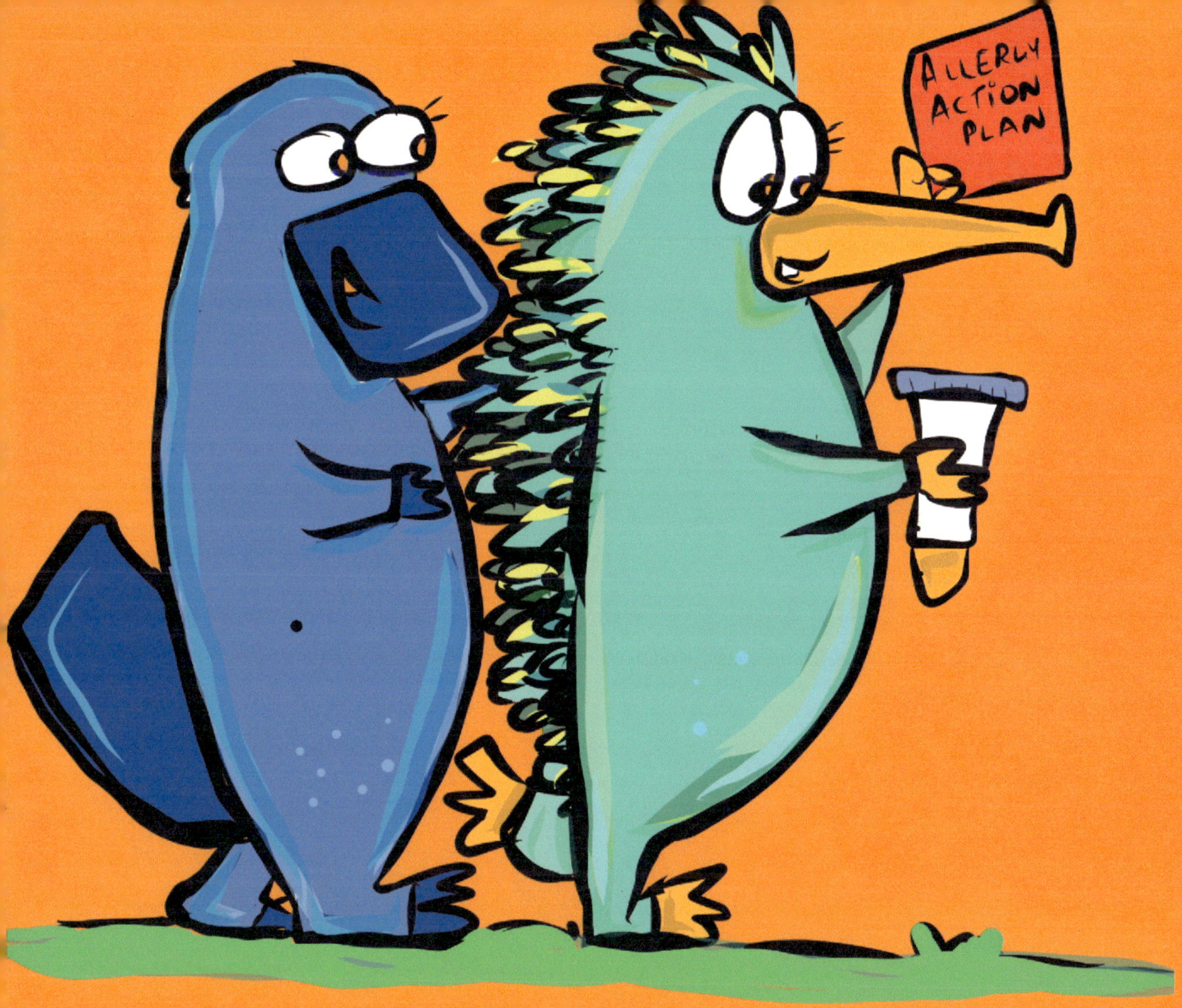

'Does your teacher at school know that you need an adrenaline pen Bobby?' asked Aiden curiously.

'My doctor did an 'ALLERGY ACTION PLAN for me so that everyone at school knows what to do if I get a bad food allergy.' replied Bobby.

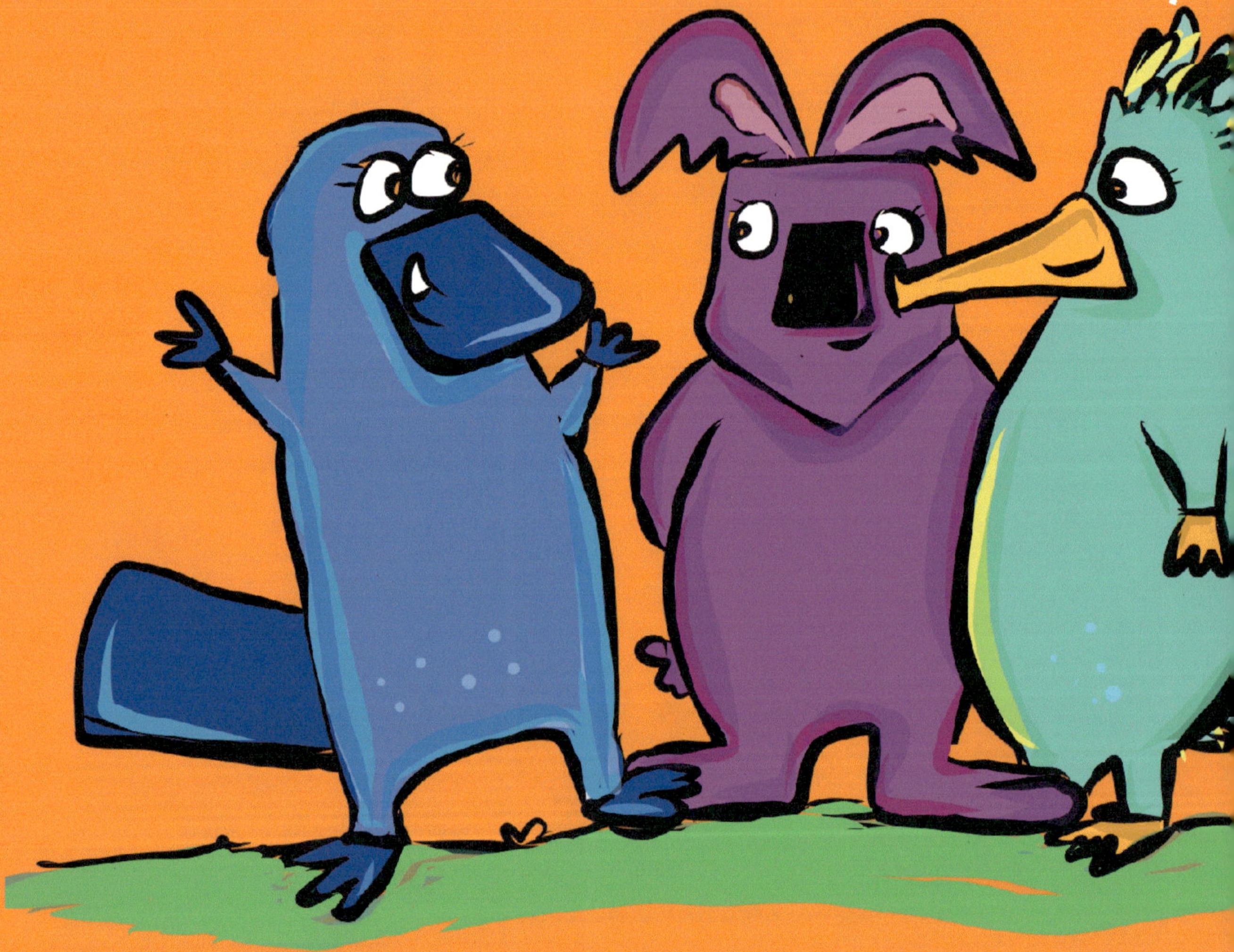

'That is great. We learnt a new lesson today to be mindful about FOOD ALLERGY!' quipped Aiden. From now on NUTS are banned from our picnics. We need to look after the health of our dear friend Bobby.' said Aiden.

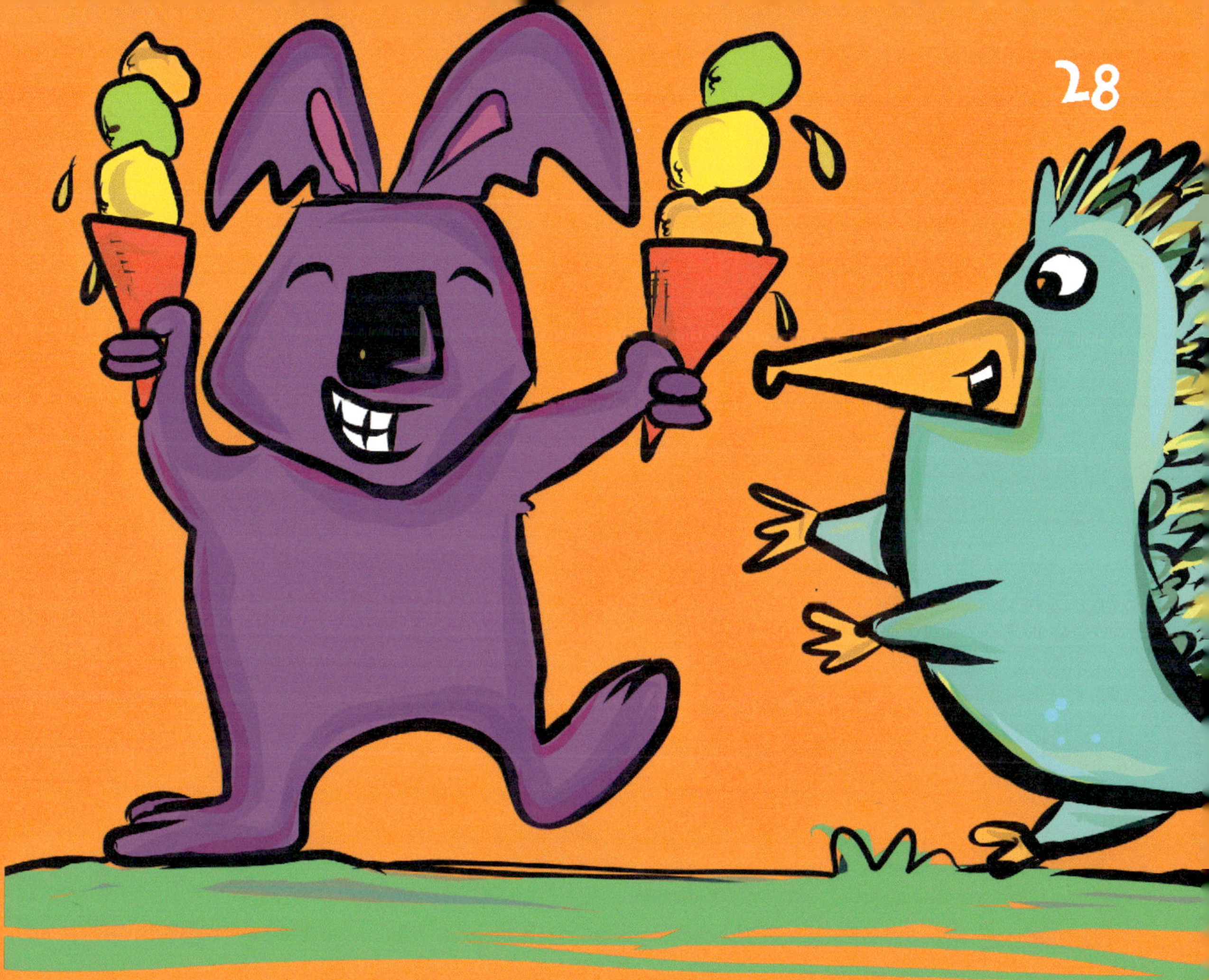

'NUT FREE' ice-creams are ready folks.' screamed Neva.

“Wait a minute, does it have cashew nuts?' asked Bobby with a big grin.

Hearing this everyone roared with laughter and ran to grab their ice-cream.

To my wonderful Neva & Aiden

First published by LIGHT AUSTRALIA in 2021.

Design and Layout by Grafixo.

ISBN 978-0-6452947-0-5

The digital illustrations of this book is created by Dr. Abraham Thomas and Neva Thomas.

Type set in Arial

Printed in Australia.

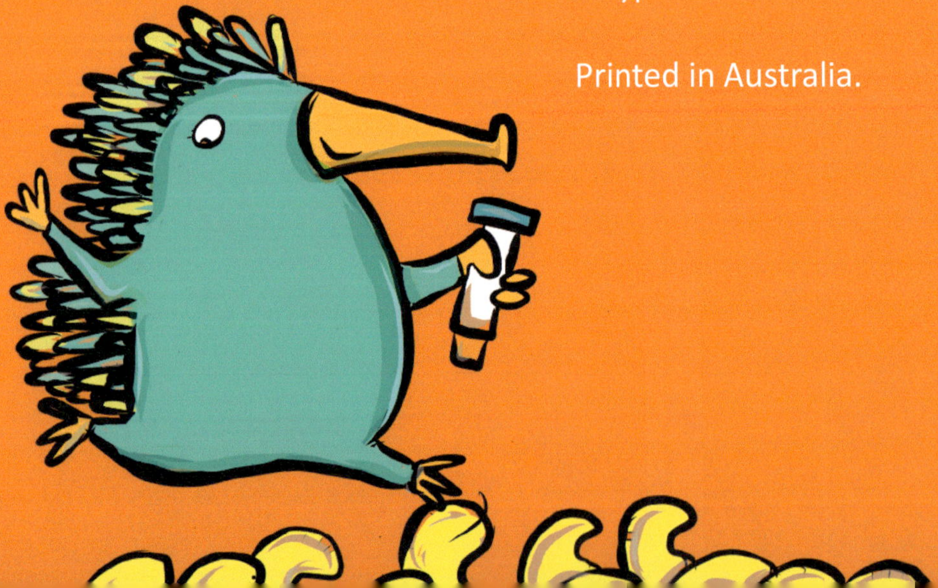

NATIONAL LIBRARY OF AUSTRALIA

A catalogue record of this book is available from the National Library of Australia

Made in the USA
Las Vegas, NV
13 November 2026

58093851R10019